STEP IT UP

BECOME YOUR OWN PERSONAL TRAINER

DR.VITO DIMATTEO, DC

IUNIVERSE, INC.
NEW YORK   BLOOMINGTON

Step It Up
become your own personal trainer

iUniverse books may be ordered through booksellers or by contacting:

iUniverse
1663 Liberty Drive
Bloomington, IN 47403
www.iuniverse.com
1-800-Authors (1-800-288-4677)

Because of the dynamic nature of the Internet, any Web addresses or links contained in this book may have changed since publication and may no longer be valid.

ISBN: 978-1-4401-1764-0 (sc)
ISBN: 978-1-4401-1765-7 (ebk)

Printed in the United States of America

iUniverse rev. date: 9/24/2009

PREFACE

This book is designed for people who need to challenge themselves on a whole new level of fitness. These exercises are designed and created to step up your current program. The exercises found in this book are modifications to current exercises, designed to challenge your fitness levels in a multidimensional approach. As a personal trainer for eight years I saw my clients grow and improve to new fitness levels. The traditional resistive training exercises were not enough. My clients insisted on being challenged. I always found the best trainers to be innovative in their program design.

I quickly began to formulate creative programs, which constantly would step up my clients fitness levels and in return a very busy schedule for me. A lot of the exercises in this book are intended for intermediate to expert fitness levels. First and foremost it is important to ensure that you have a strong foundation in exercise, form and body awareness. It is important for people to be aware of their body and control over their movements. Secondly, I focus on core strength. It is essential to have a strong core so that major muscles of the body can grow in size and strength. For example, the multifidi, rotators and intertraversi muscles are all muscles that surround the spine and lay the foundation for a strong core.

There is no other book out there that offers what I have composed. I have documented some of the most challenging exercises that I have used to step up my clients workouts.

ACKNOWLEDGMENTS

I would like to extend a special thanks to my dear friend Alex Arrieta, the best photographer I know for taking time out of his busy schedule to capture the focus of each exercise. I would also like to thank the models for donating their time and efforts the help create this exercise book. Last but not least, I would like to extend a special thanks to my wife Monica. Without her support and encouragement this book would never be possible. This book is dedicated to my beautiful daughter Isabella Mia. Who showed me what life is all about. Daddy loves you.

One Legged Hungarian Dead Lift.

This exercise is very challenging it will work on your unilateral balance, and the ability to move while stabilizing. It will incorporate upper and lower body muscles, making it a very functional exercise. Major Muscle groups utilized here are abdominals, spinal erectors, biceps, and the glutes.

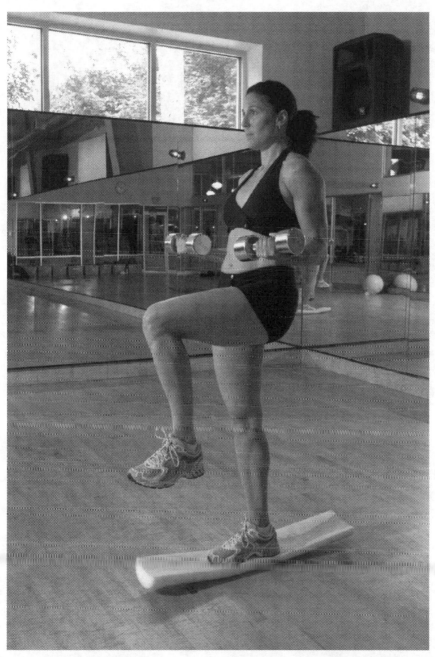

1a: Start off balancing on one leg as shown; the balance foam is used to add difficulty. Flex the non weight bearing leg, and curl the dumbbells, preferably a weight which you can normally curl for 15 reps.

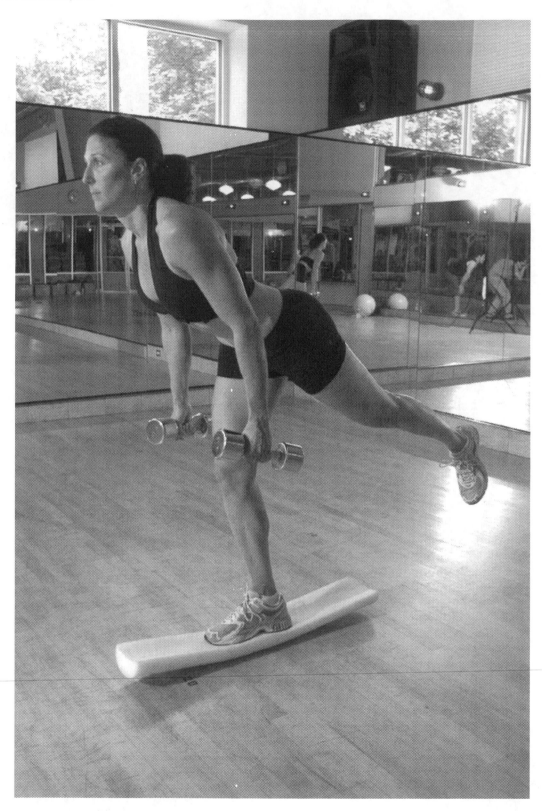

1b: Begin to lower your body by flexing at the stabilizing hip (weight bearing leg) at the same time lower your arms toward the ground and kick the non-stabilizing hip (non weight bearing leg) into extension.

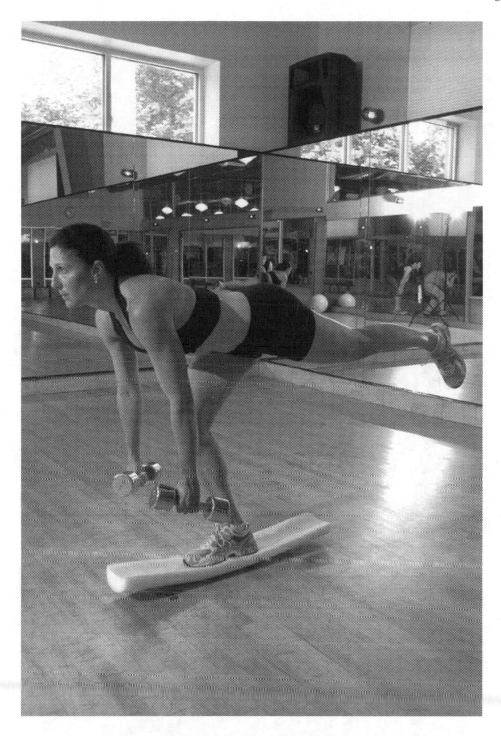

1c: Try to make your self parallel to the ground, hold for 2 seconds, and then slowly do the reverse returning yourself to the starting position. Movements are always most effective when performed slowly and controlled. Number of repetitions is up to you, I always aim for 10 on each side.

Tip: Focusing on an object helps in maintaining your balance.

One Legged Ball Squats

This exercise will focus on your ability to stabilize and at the same time isolating the deep fibers of the gluteus maximus. This is also a functional exercise utilizing upper and lower body muscles. The major muscles used are glute maximus, hamstrings, quadriceps, core abdominals, and the shoulder deltoid group.

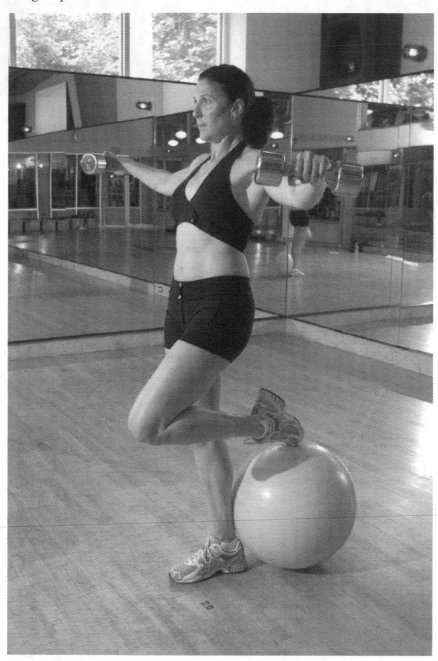

2a: Start the exercise stabilizing on the ball (ball should be about knee height as shown) with the non weight bearing leg, perform a lateral raise utilizing a weight that you can lift for 15 reps.

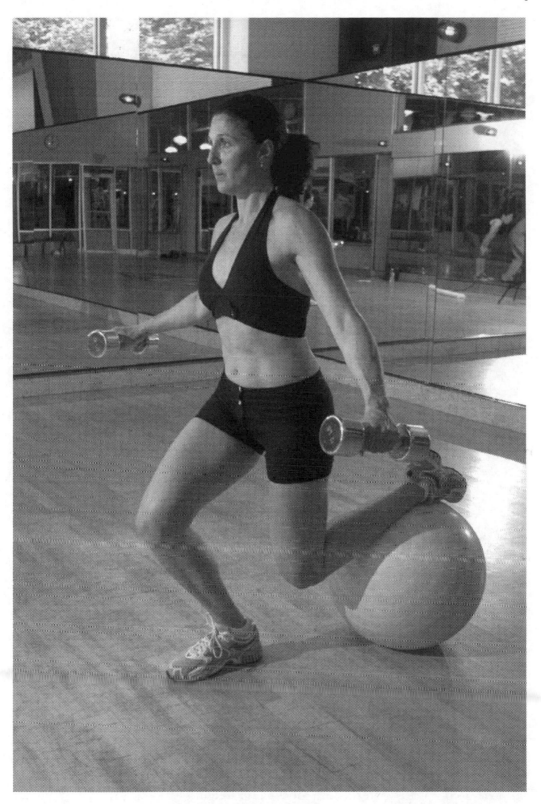

2b: Begin to lower your hips with your arms by bending at the knee of the weight bearing leg. The trick here is to lower your butt into the direction of the ball while driving the non-weight bearing knee into the ground.

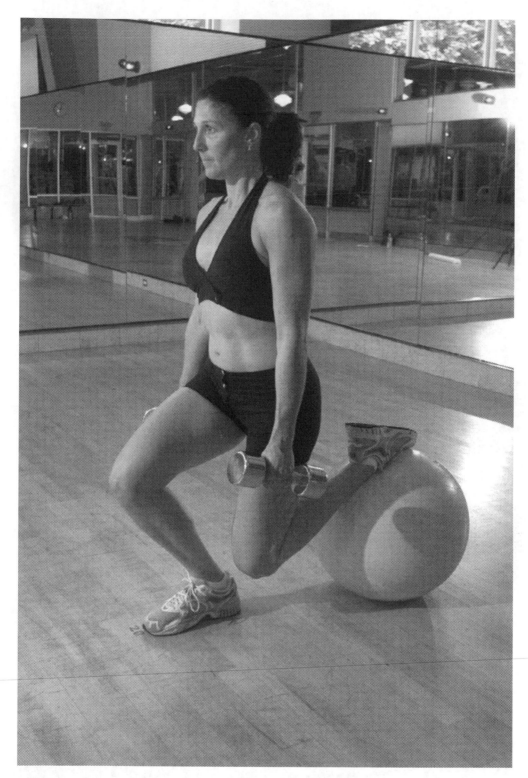

2c: The move is complete when the knee of the non weight bearing leg is about 5 inches from the ground.

Tip: This is also a good way to dynamically stretch your quads. Remember to focus on an object to assist in balance.

Push Up Crossovers.

This exercise will challenge your ability to maintain a tight stable core at the same time deeply isolating the pectoral fibers.

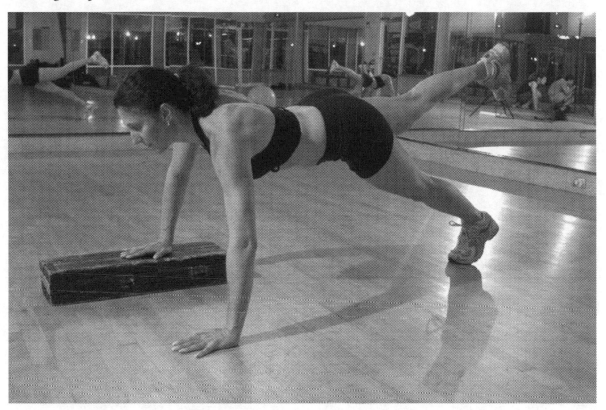

3a: Choose a step that is approximately 4-5in. The larger the height, the more difficult it is. Be sure to maintain a 60 degree angle from elbow to the rib cage. Keep a tight stomach and lower yourself until a good stretch is felt in the pectoral fibers.

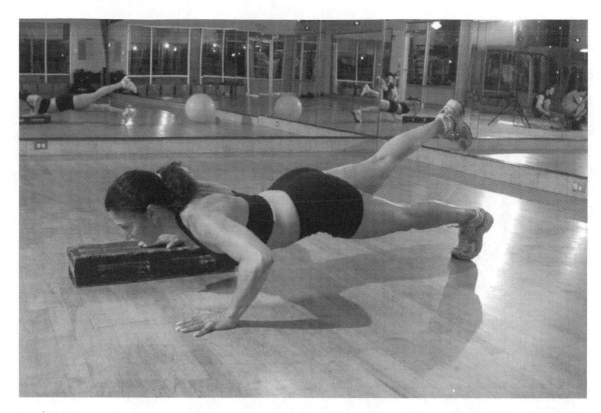

3b: Try to suck in the naval; maintaining a tight core.

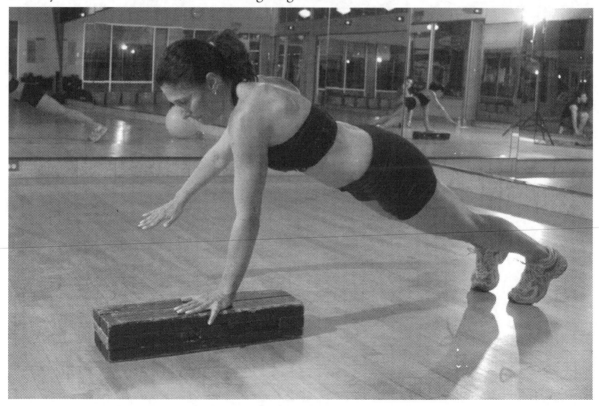

3c: Come out of the push up beginning to cross over. At this point switch feet and arms, and lower yourself down into a push up as shown in 3d.

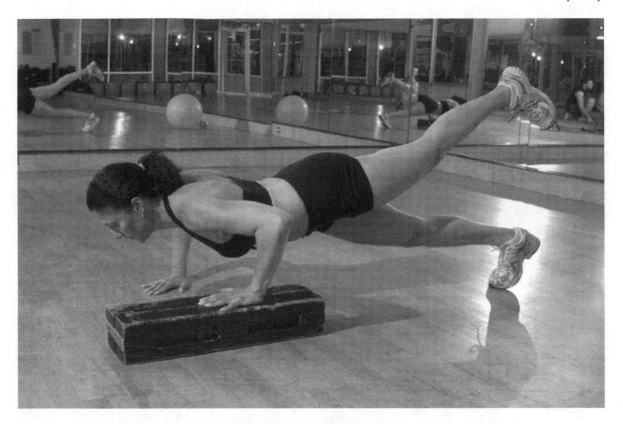

Tip: If crossing over is too much of a challenge at this point, remain on the same side for 5-7 reps then move over to the other side.

Half Foam Squat With Ball Toss.

This exercise is best performed with a partner. If a partner is not available, you may also throw the ball into an upright mini-trampoline. Your ability to balance and maintain stability is challenged in a multiplanar aspect.

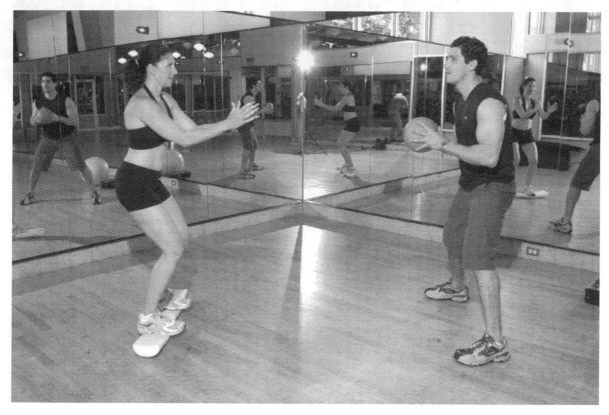

4a: The half foam will assist you in performing a perfect squat, falling off the edges signifies poor form. Catch the ball at the top of the motion (choose a ball weight that you can handle) hold and squat. Once you're in a full squat throw the ball back as shown in picture 4c.
Repeat the movement for 10-15 reps.

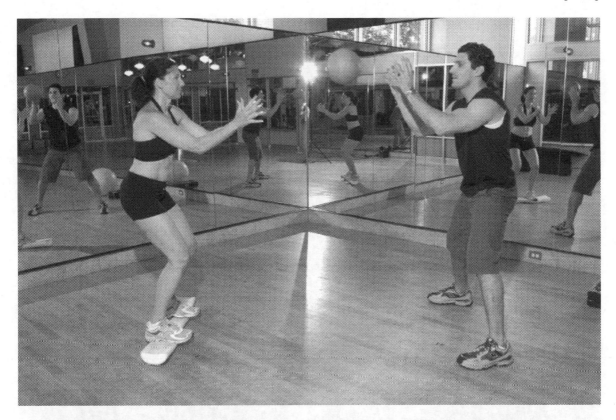

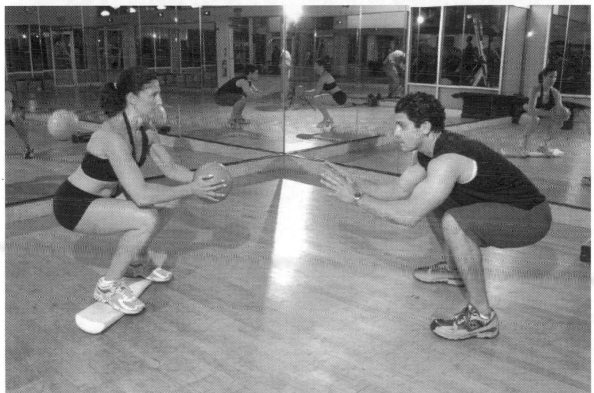

Tip: Perform the squat first until you are comfortable, and then utilize the ball.

Ball Knee To Chest Push Ups.

This exercise will challenge the abdominal muscles, as well as the upper pectoral group and anterior deltoids.

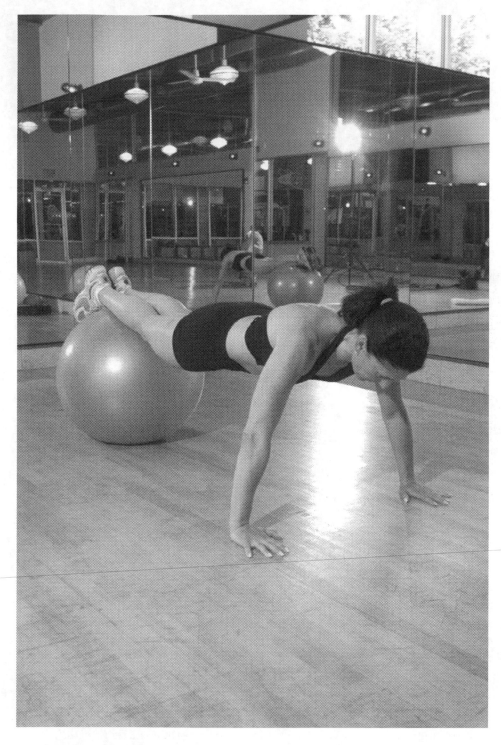

5a: Start by holding the bridge position, feet and legs tightly together and elbows slightly bent.

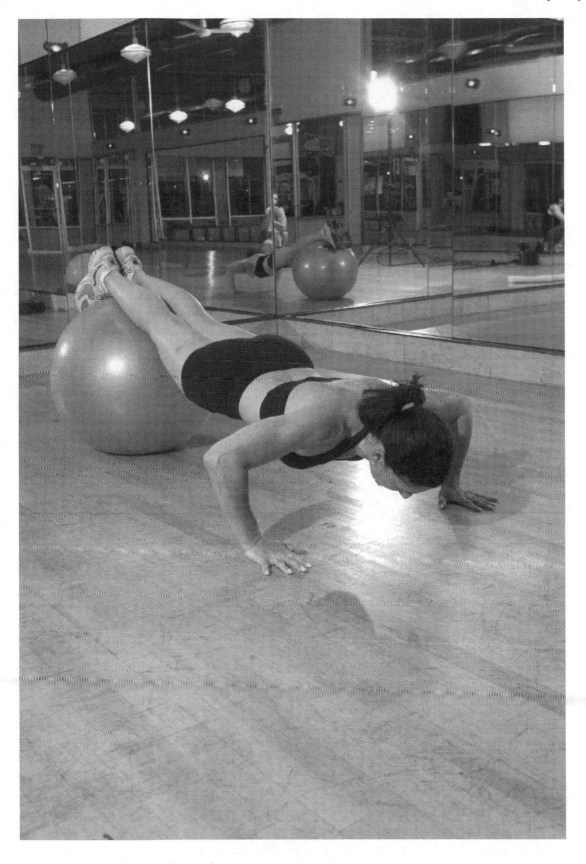

5b: Lower your body into the push up.

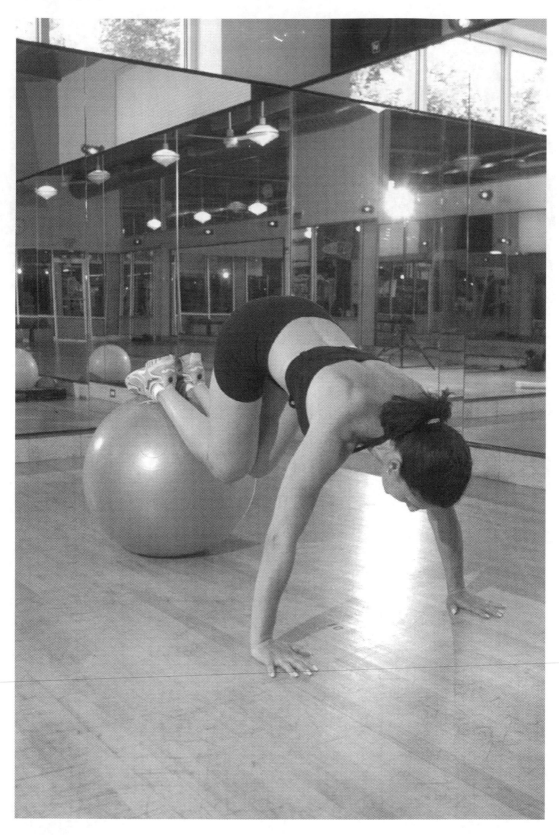

5c: Push yourself up and at the same time initiate the knee tuck to the chest. Hold at end range for a count of 3 seconds. Then end by returning to the bridge.

One Legged Ball Knee To Chest Push Ups.

This exercise is a step up from the bilateral knee to chest exercise. It will force you to isolate the external and internal oblique region.

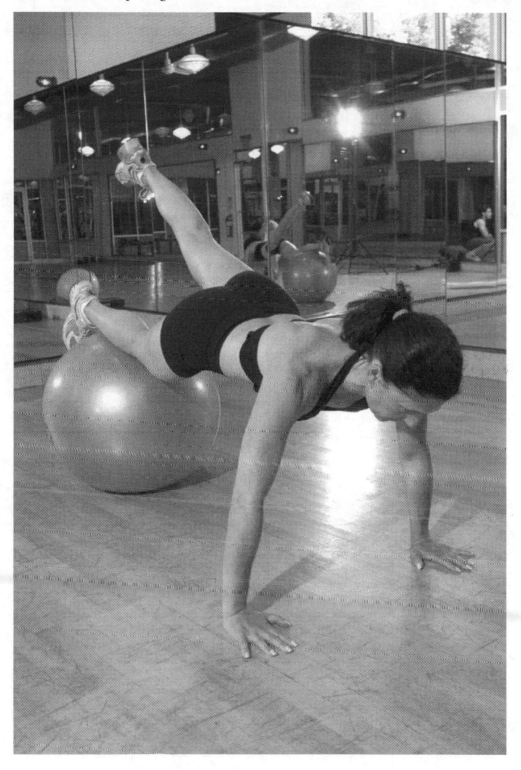

6a: Start the exercise in the bridge position with one leg up.

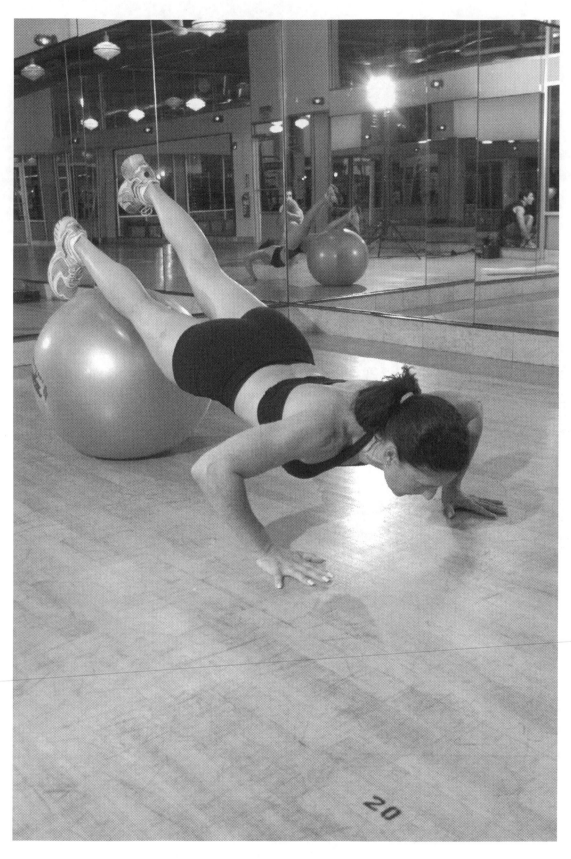

6b: From the bridge position proceed to go into a push up.

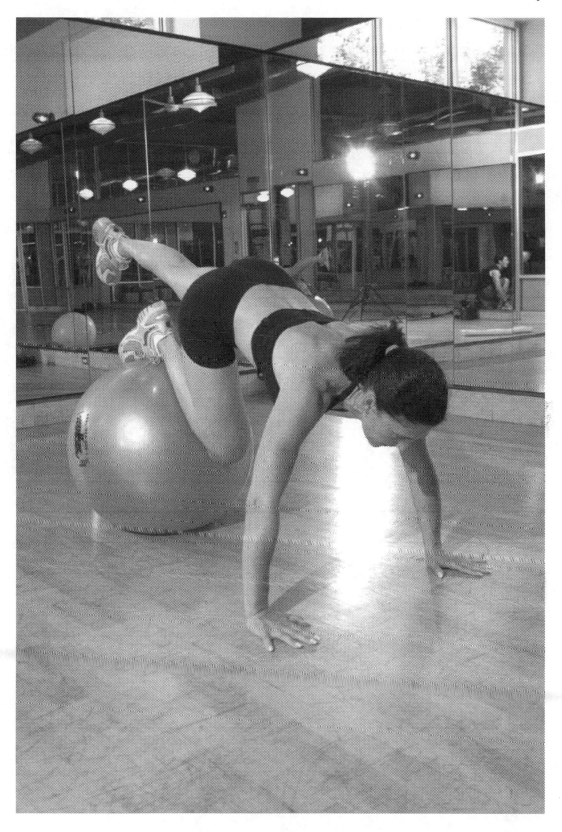

6c: As you ascend from the push up position begin to follow up with the stabilizing leg by pulling it into your chest.

Supine One Legged Ball Bridge.

This exercise is a good way to improve your balance while isolating the gluteus region, hamstrings, and abdominals.

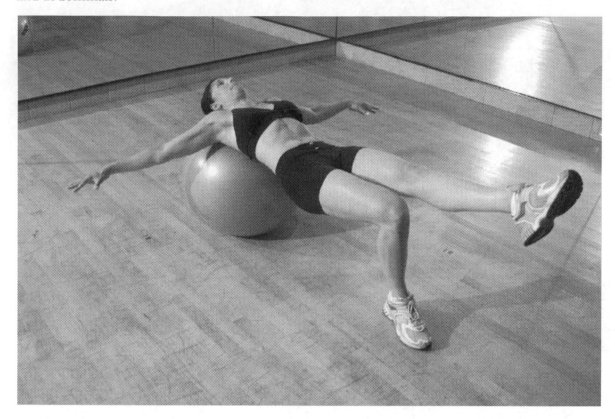

7a: Position yourself on the ball as shown in the picture. Be sure to maintain a tight core and initially avoid letting your pelvis drop to the ground.

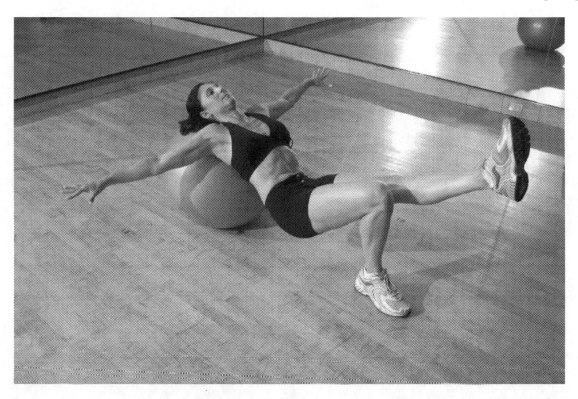

7b: Lower your pelvis a few inches from the ground while maintaining your balance on the ball.

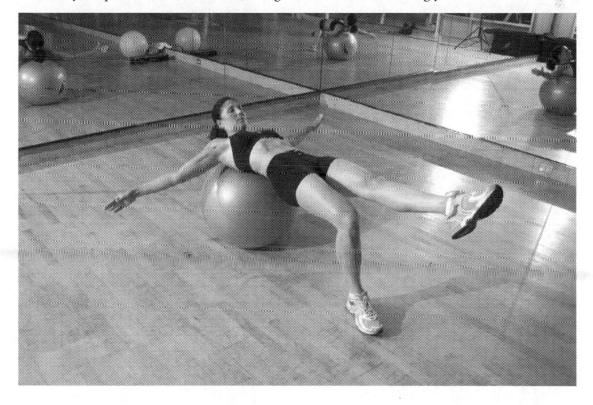

7c: To really feel the effects of this exercise focus on pushing the pelvis up to the ceiling while contracting the glutes.

Step Push Ups With Side Bridge.

This exercise will focus on your ability to maintain stability while transitioning into a new movement.

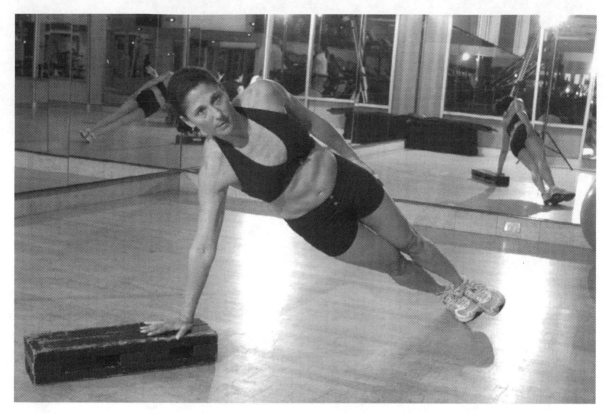

8a: Start the exercise in a sideways bridge. Be sure to hold a tight core and keep the body in a straight line.

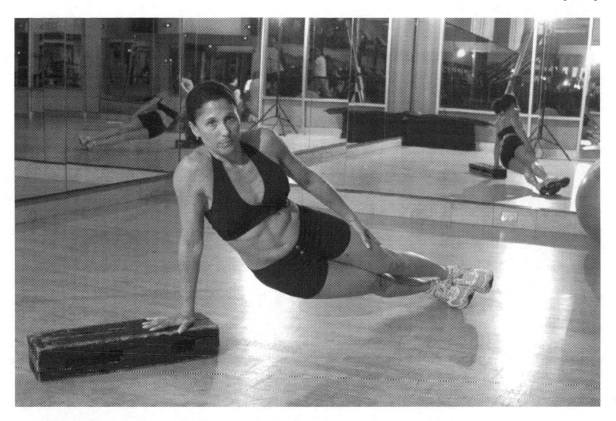

8b: Lower your pelvis to the ground until a stretch is felt on the lower side.

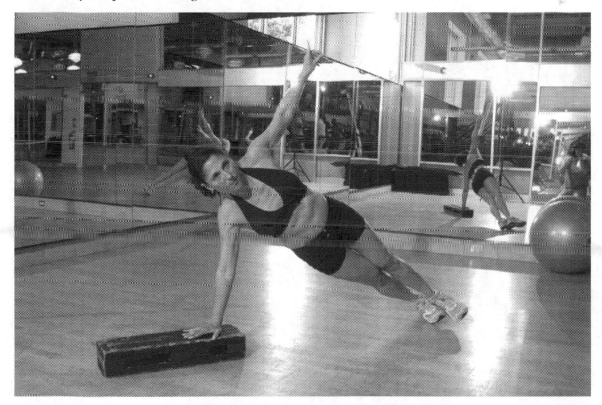

8c: Return to the bridge position feeling the oblique muscle group working.

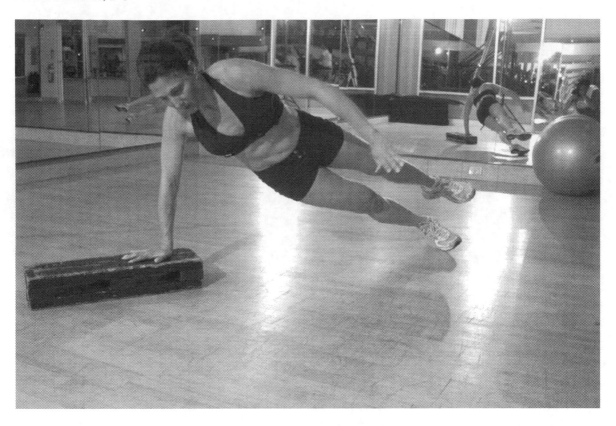

8d: To further challenge yourself, in the bridge position begin to lower yourself into a push-up as shown in the next illustration.

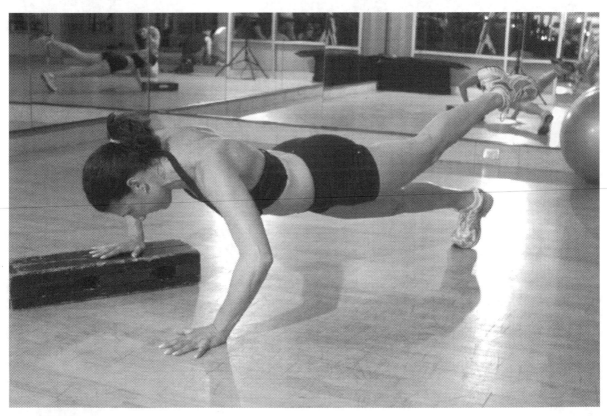

One Legged Dumbbell Ball Press Ups.

This exercise will be a great step up from the traditional bench press.

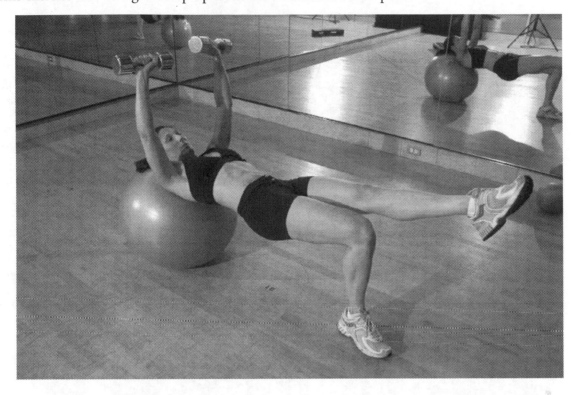

9a: Begin with a ball bridge with one leg up. Then proceed with a dumbbell press up as shown in the following illustration.

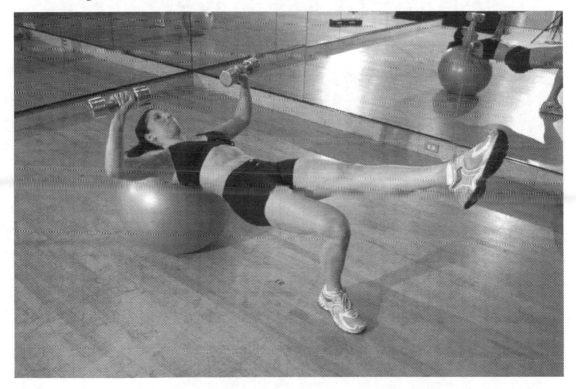

Half Foam Squat Thrust.

This is a full body exercise which will increase your heart rate! It is a great way to warm up.

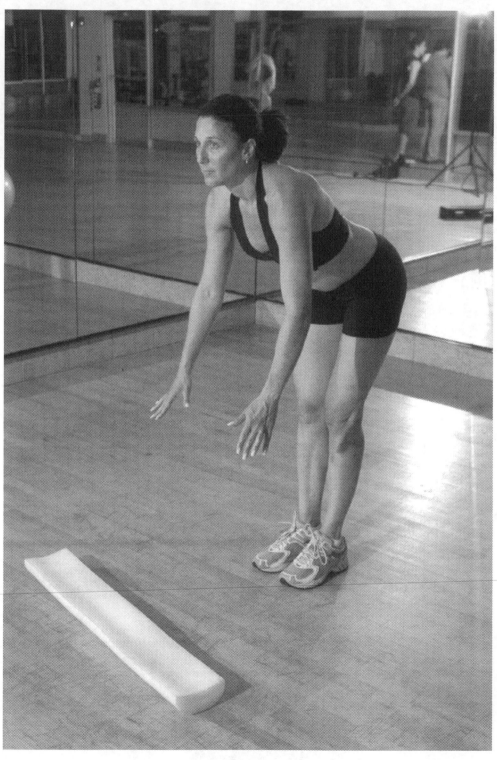

10a: Start in the upright position with a slight bend at the hips.

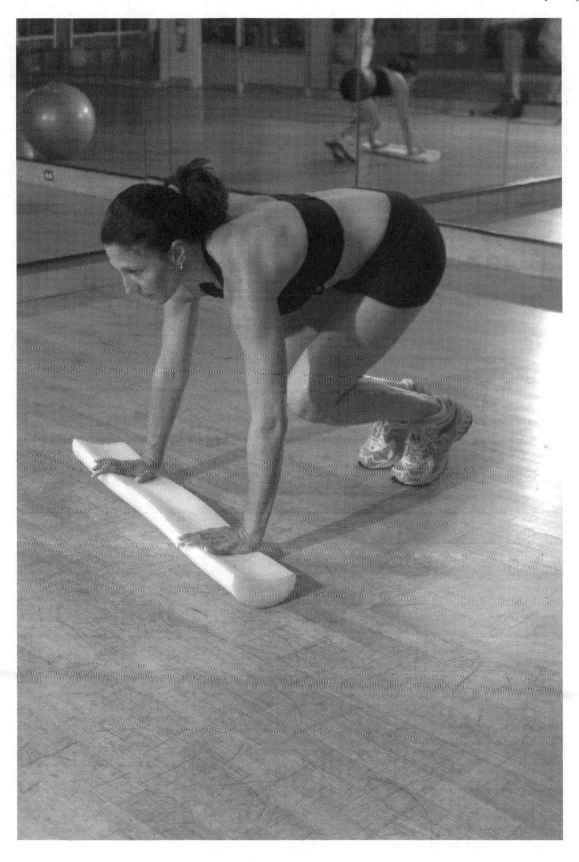

10b.

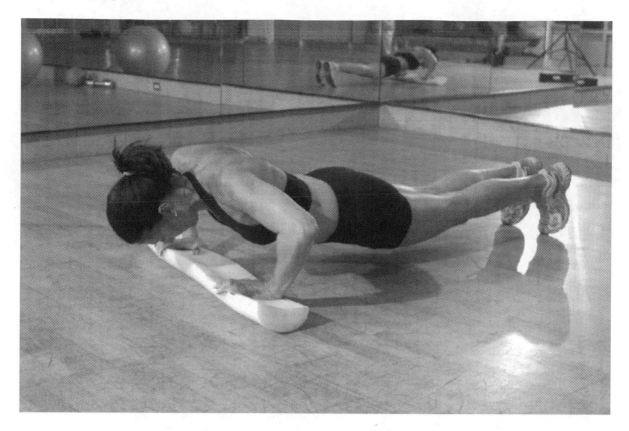

10c: Drop into the push-up position trying to maintain balance on the half foam log.

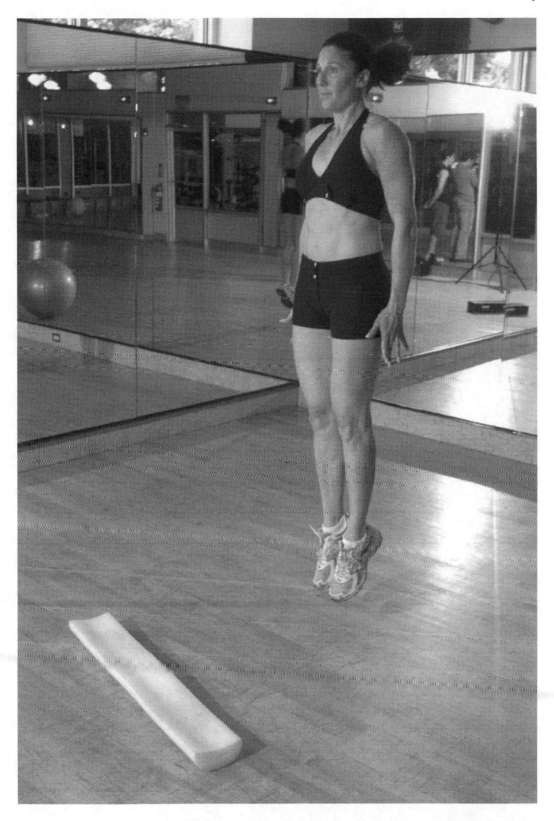

10d: Once the push-up is complete challenge yourself by exploding up into the air and returning back down to the upright position.

Trampoline Sprints.

This exercise helps develop your speed and increase your endurance without the impact.

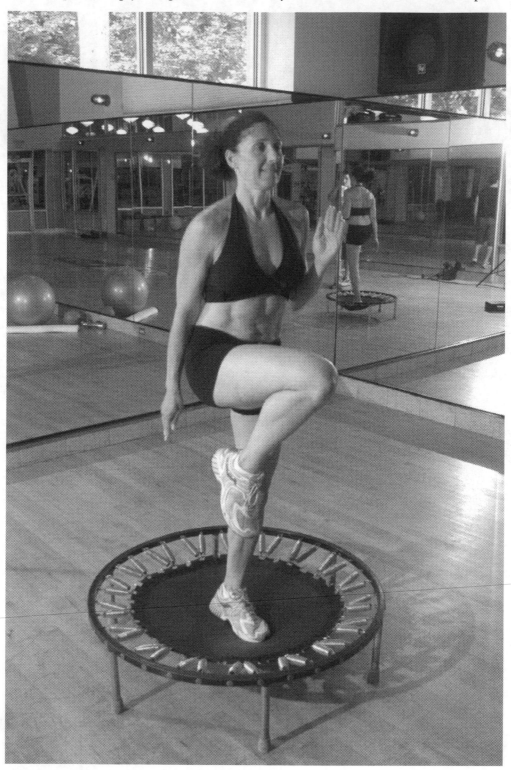

11a: Be sure to maintain your body position centered on the trampoline while sprinting in place.

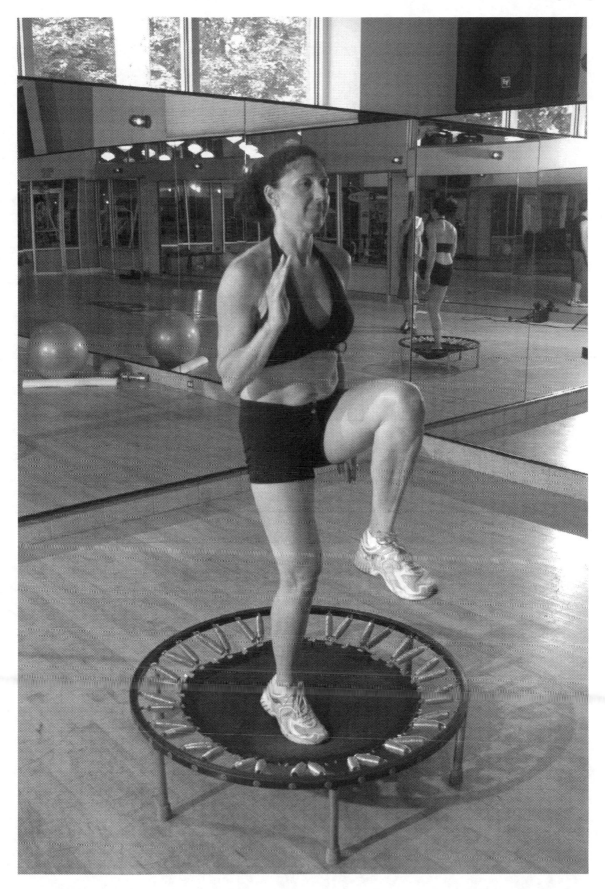

Trampoline Mogul Sprints.

This is a great way to improve your strength and coordination when attacking the moguls on the slopes. For those of you who do not ski, this exercise will give you a great abdominal workout.

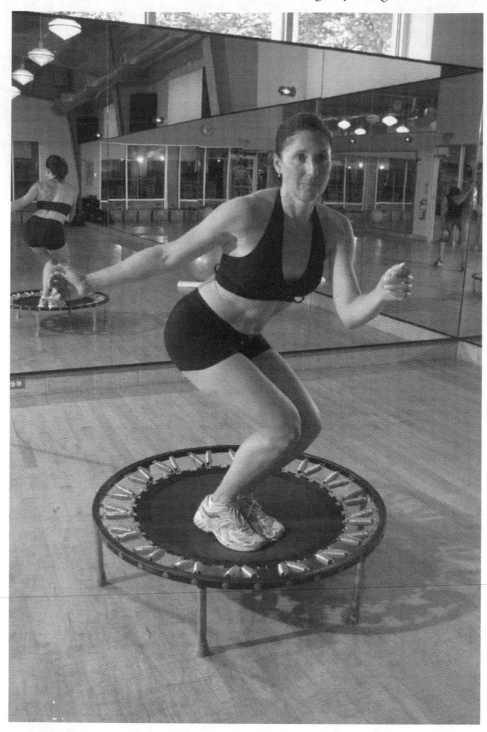

12a: Start to one side keeping the knees bent and together.

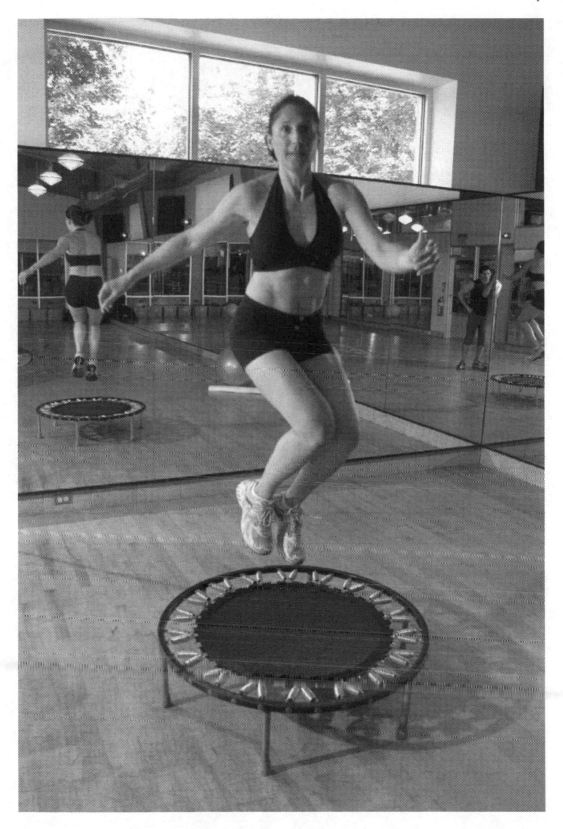

12b: When crossing over to the other side be sure to keep the legs together pulling the knees in. Most of the power must be generated by the abdominal muscles.

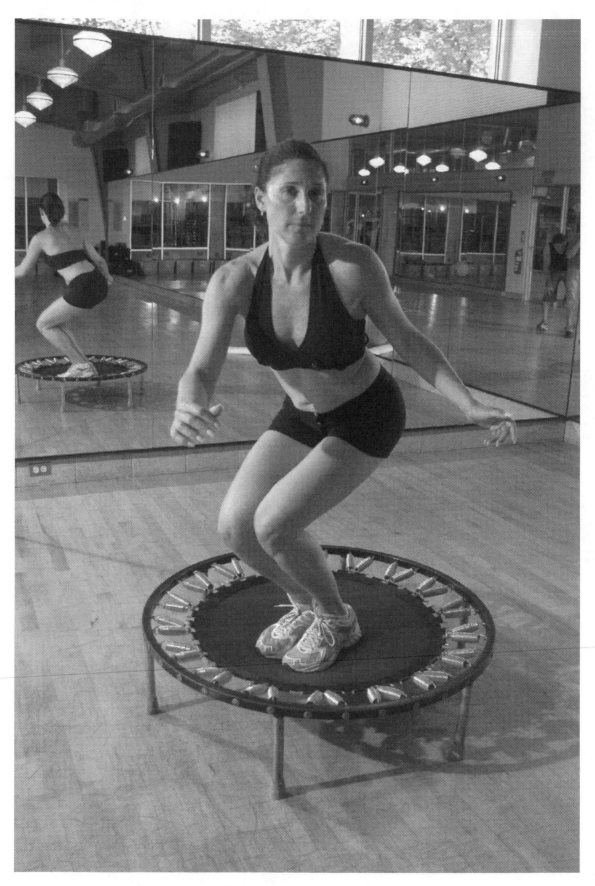

Trampoline 180 Degree Jumps.

This exercise is great for the extreme skier and snowboarder. It will challenge your ability to change direction in mid air.

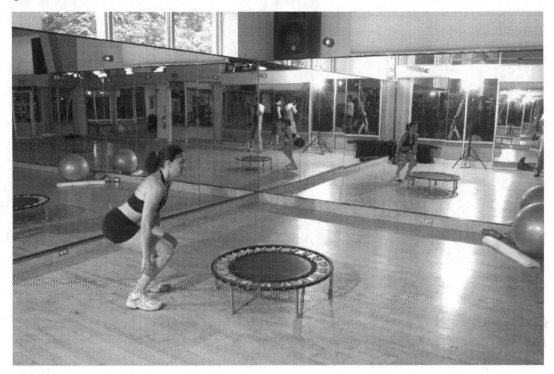

13a: Start the exercise in semi-squat position; explode upwards and jump onto the trampoline as shown in picture 13b.

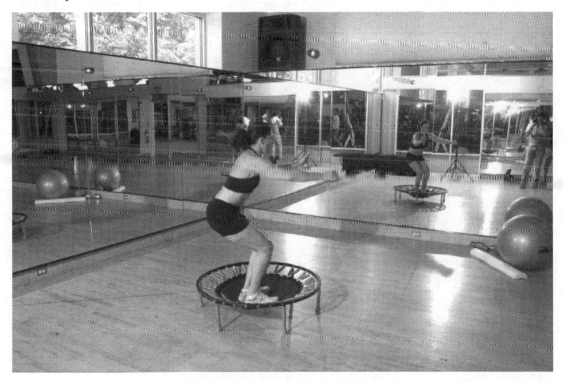

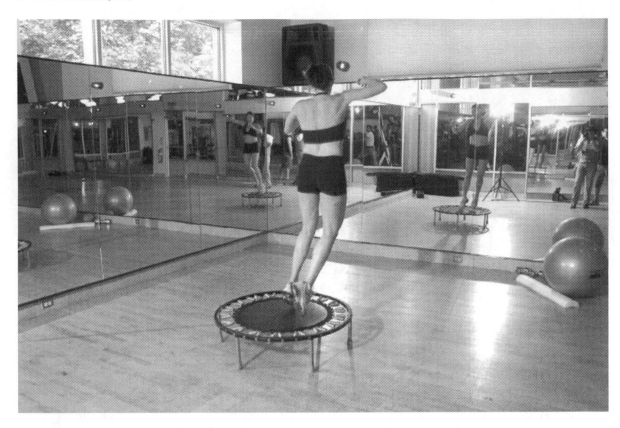

13c: When jumping off the trampoline begin to spin half way around, 180 degrees, land facing the trampoline as shown in figure 13d.

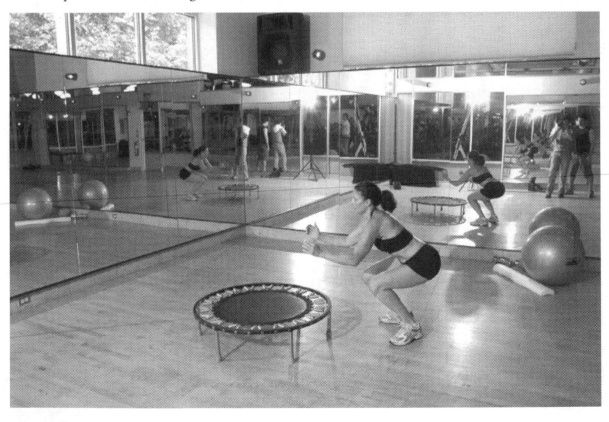

Trampoline Sideway Jumps.

This exercise will require you to turn 180 degrees before reaching the trampoline.

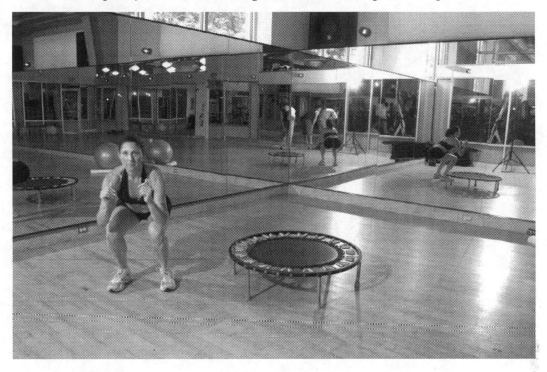

14a: Start in the squatted position. When jumping, begin to rotate towards the trampoline.

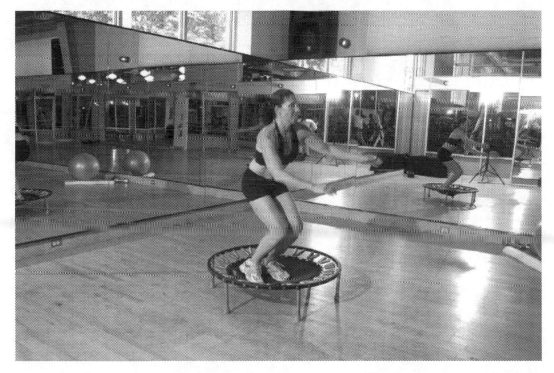

14b: When landing on the trampoline, go into a squat and jump off sideways facing the other direction as shown in picture 14c.

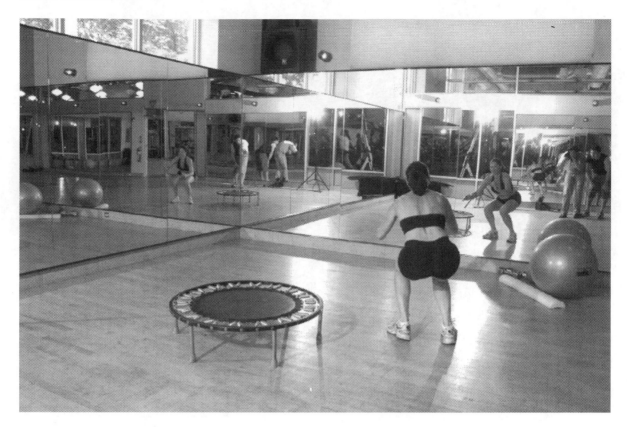

14c.

Medicine Ball Sideways Trampoline Jumps.

This exercise requires the help of a partner. It requires explosive speed and agility. Start off slow going through the movement to develop perception of the surrounding space.

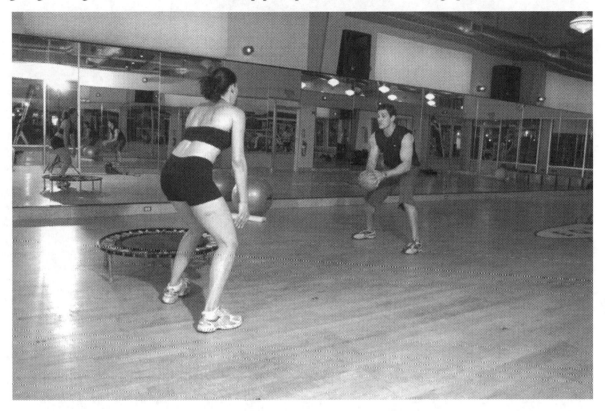

15a: Start in the squatted position and keep your abdominals tight to protect the lower back.

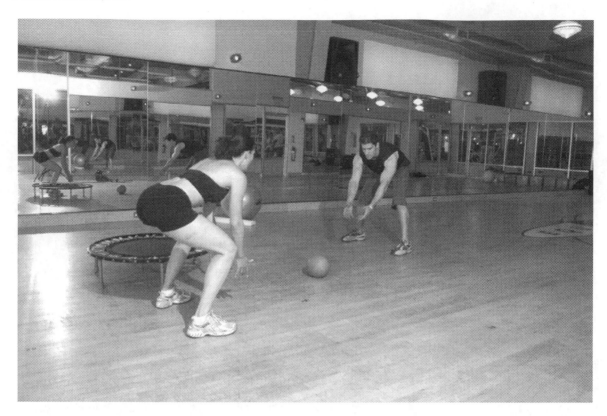

15b: The medicine ball is rolled to you.

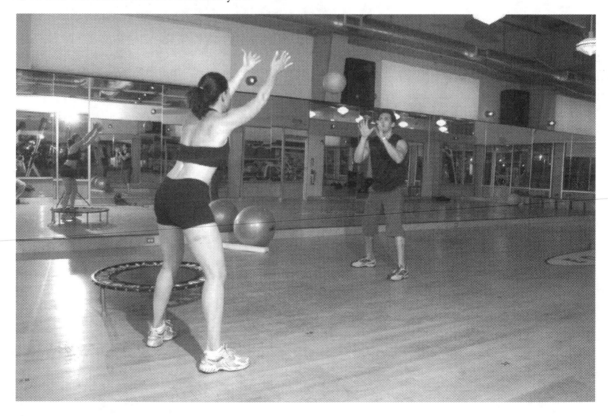

15c: Pick it up and throw it back as shown in this picture.

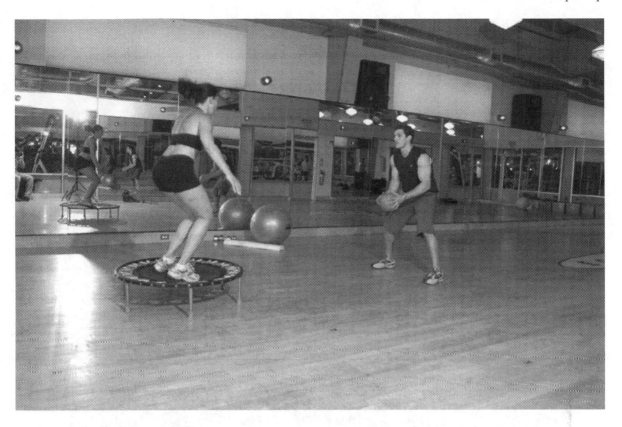

15d: Once the ball is thrown, begin to jump onto the trampoline sideways as shown in 15d. Be prepared to repeat this on the other side.

One Legged Ball Wall Squats.

One legged squats help isolate the glutel and quadriceps muscle groups.

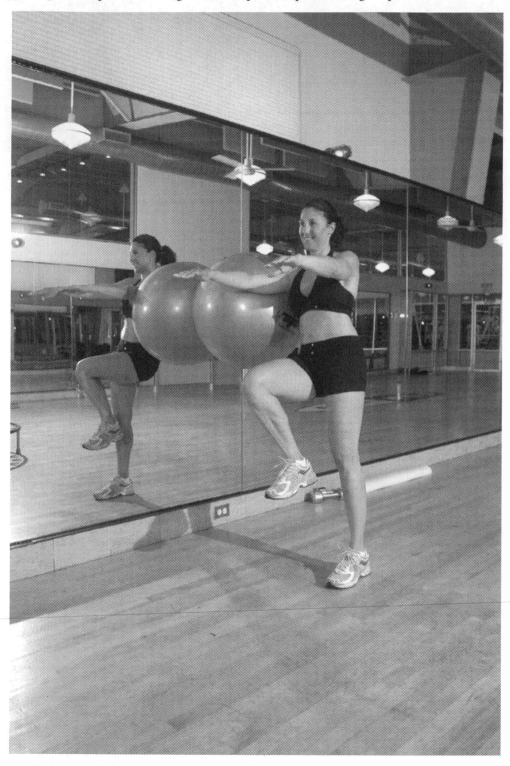

16a: When performing this exercise, lean into the ball about 30 percent of your body weight as shown in 16a.

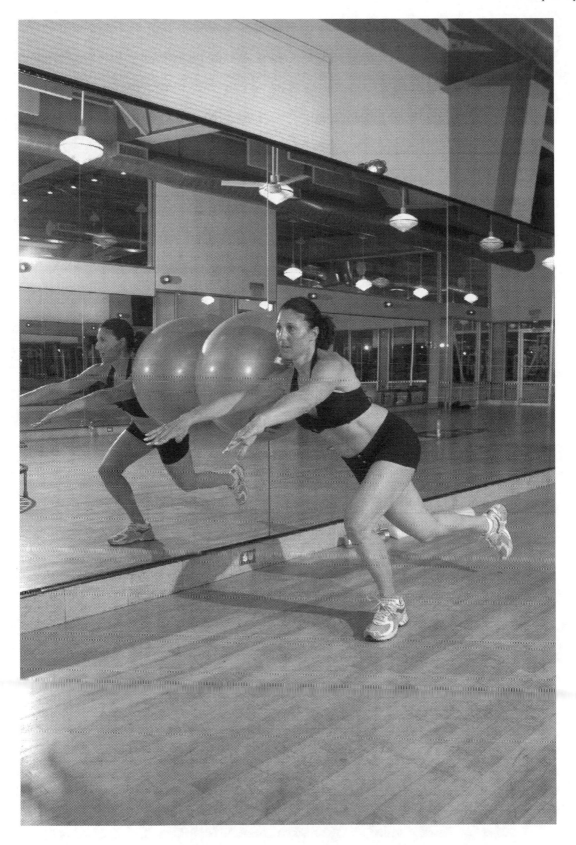

16b: Then begin to lower yourself with the leg that's furthest away from the wall.

Foam Roll Cable Crunches.

At some time or another, we all have tried cable crunches. But in order to really isolate the abdominal region, you must lock in the lower extremities with the foam roll which promotes good form.

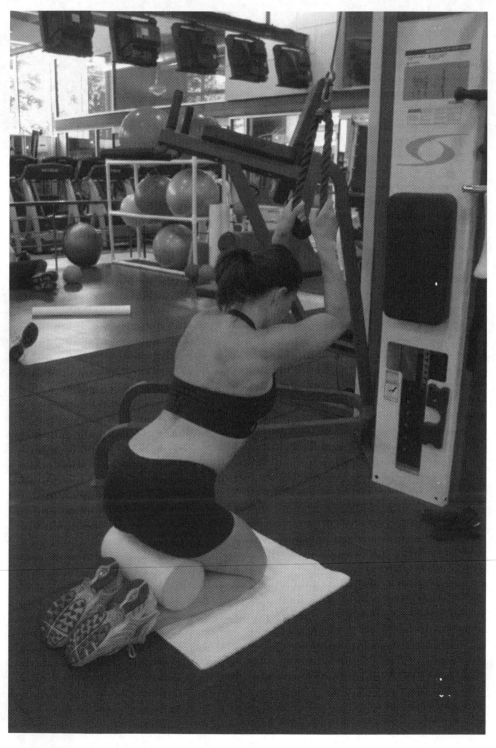

17a: The foam roll goes in between the glutes and heels as shown in 17a.

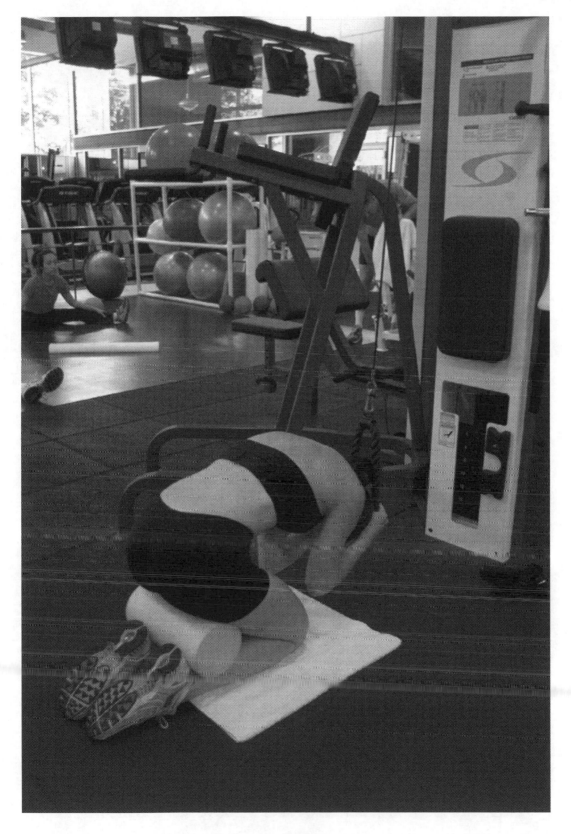

17b: Sit back onto the foam roll and begin to crunch.

Controlled slow movements are always most effective for the abdominals.

Cable Bridge Pull.

Wow, this exercise is definitely not for beginners. If you really want to challenge your core, than this is how!

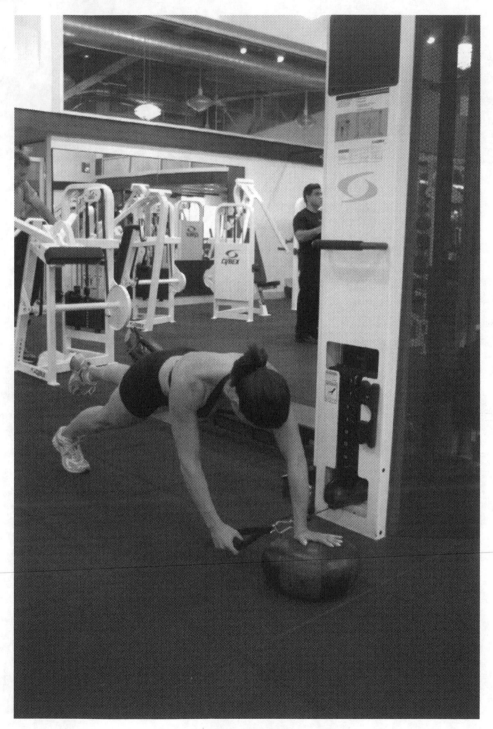

18a: Start the exercise in the planked position and maintain a strong and stable core, as shown in this picture.

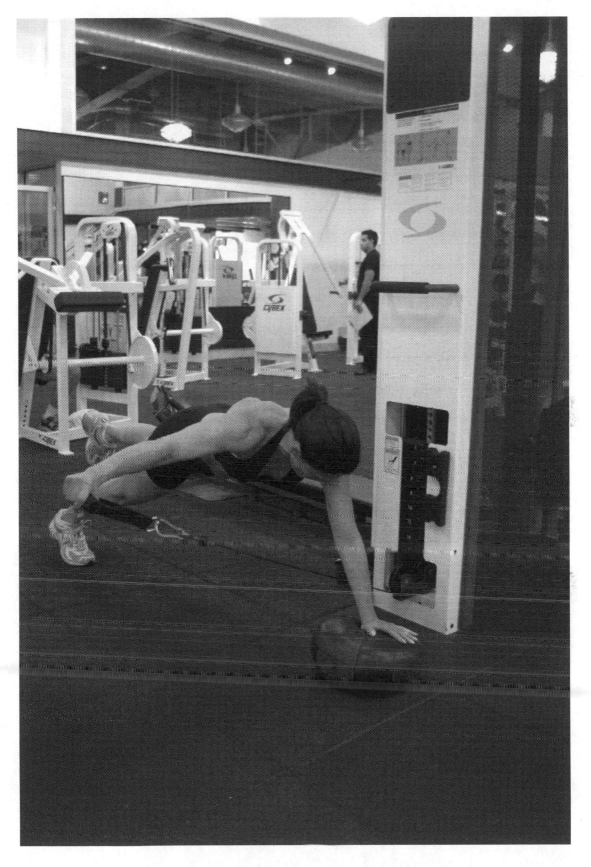

18b: Lift the opposite leg from the arm that is moving the cable.

Cable Backwards Lunge.
This exercise combines upper and lower body movements; increasing the heart rate and expediting greater calories.

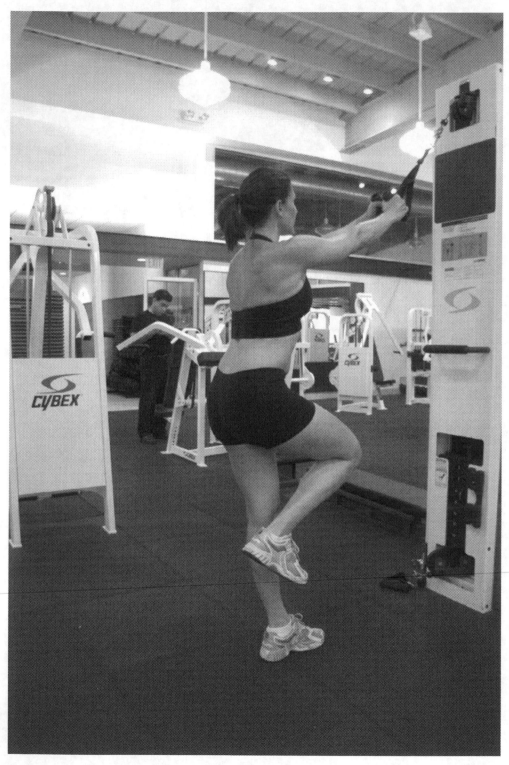

19a: Start in an upright position.

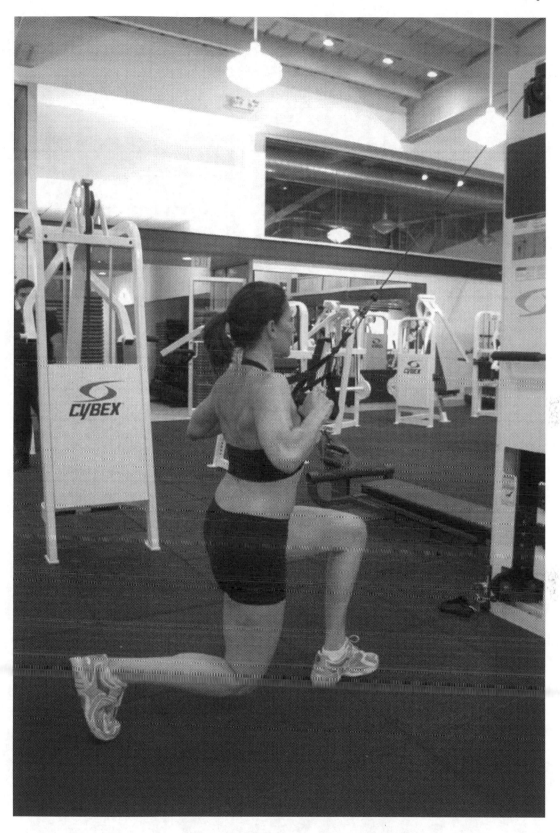

19b: Begin to lunge backwards while at the same time, pulling in the elbows into a cable row as shown in this picture.

Abdominal Ball Leg Lifts.

This exercise will challenge your ability to stabilize on the ball while performing straight leg raises.

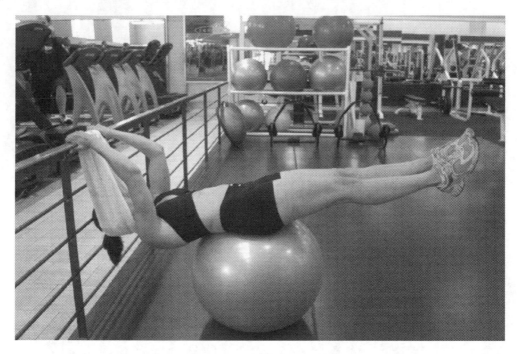

20a: Begin with finding an area that you can anchor your arms onto for increased stability. Use a towel to harness your head so the neck musculature is not overly worked; however, this is not mandatory.

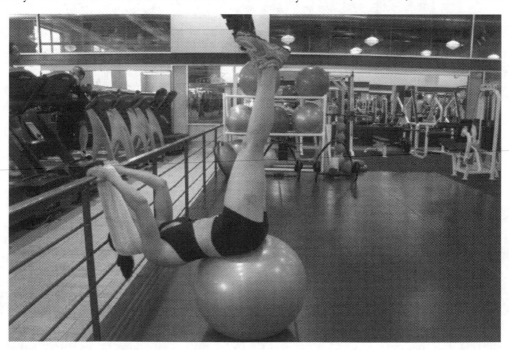

20b: Once stable on the ball begin to initiate leg movement as shown here.

One Legged Half Foam Squat.

This exercise is a great way to isolate your squatting muscles unilaterally. This will help improve your one legged balancing while also strengthening.

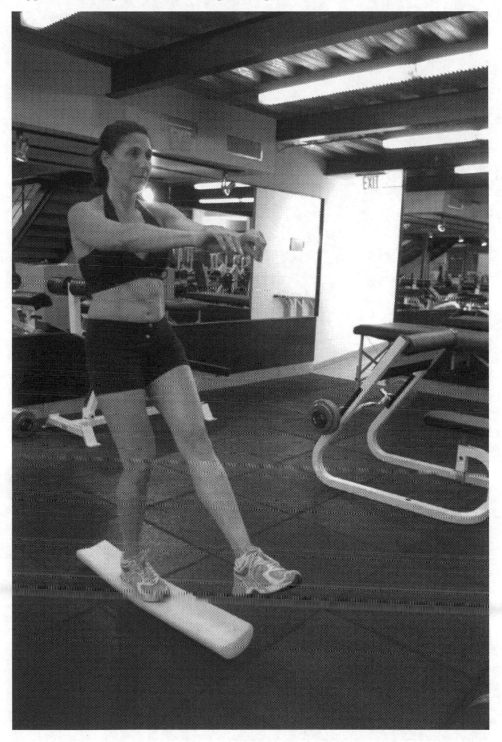

21a: Begin by standing on the half foam roll. Once you feel comfortable and balanced, initiate the squatting motion.

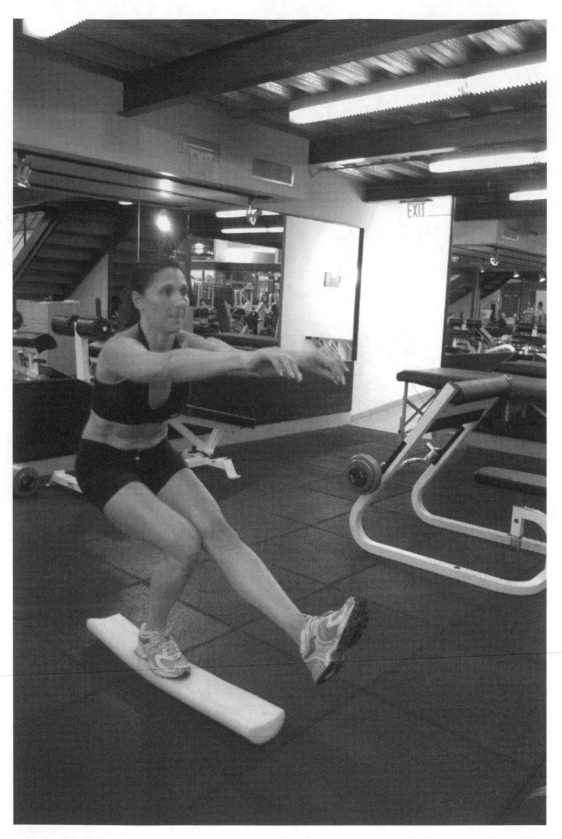

21b: It is important to hold a strong core and to move slowly as shown in picture 21B. This exercise will create fatigue within the glutes.

Dumbbell Press Squats.

This exercise combines upper and lower body muscles, increasing the heart rate and therefore burning more calories. This is another great way to warm up.

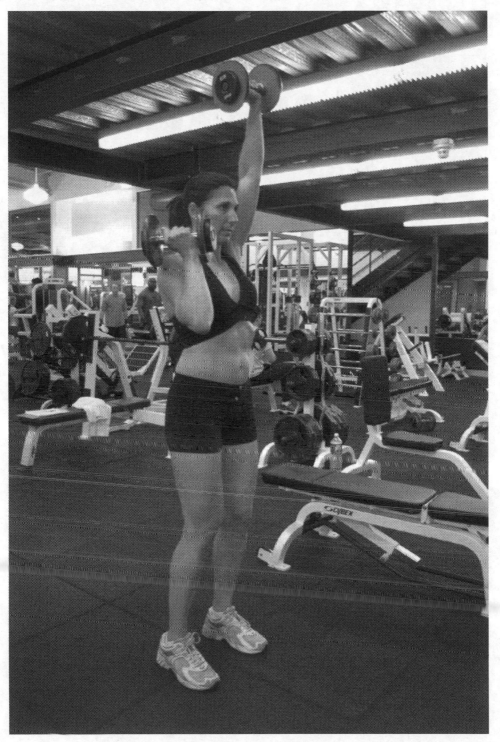

22a: Start the exercise with a comfortable weight that you can do high reps with. Slightly bend the knees as shown in this picture.

Begin to press alternating arms in-between squats as shown in 22b and 22c.

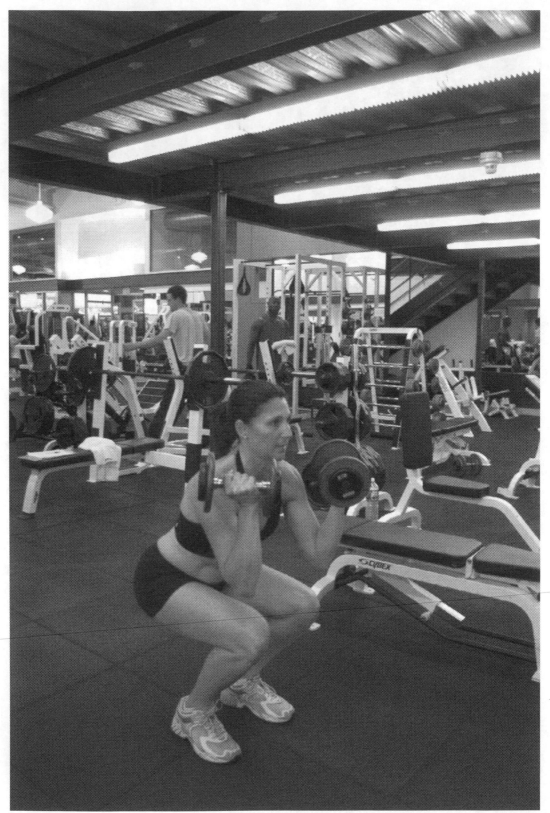

22b:

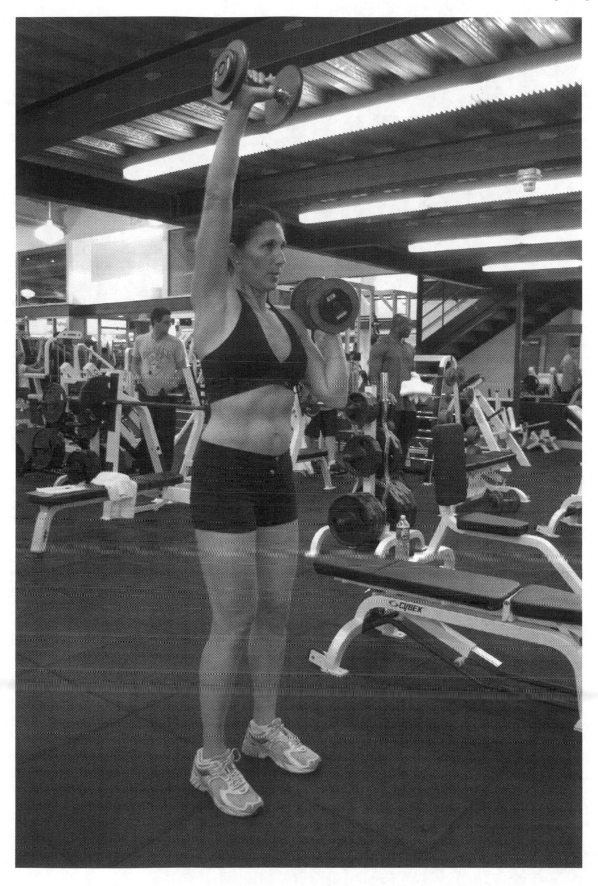

One Legged Up-Right Dumbbell Row.

This exercise is a great way to target the shoulder musculature without the harmful effects of the standard up-right row. Indirectly it will also focus on the abdominal musculature.

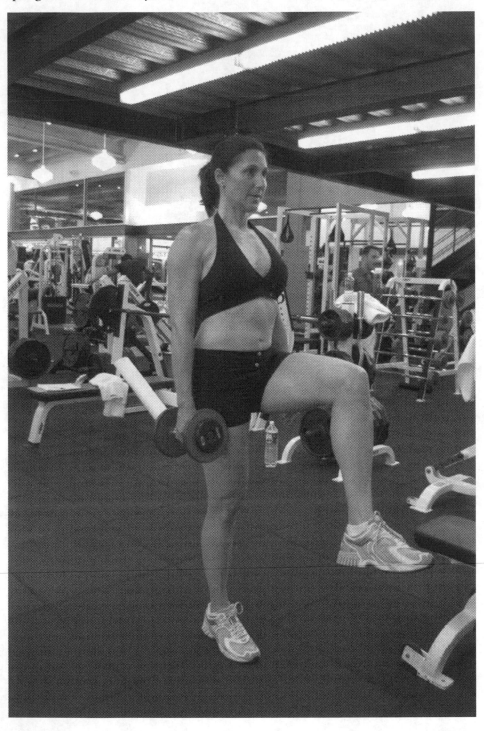

Begin the exercise by balancing on one leg, the opposite leg of the shoulder in training is recommended as shown in figure 23A.

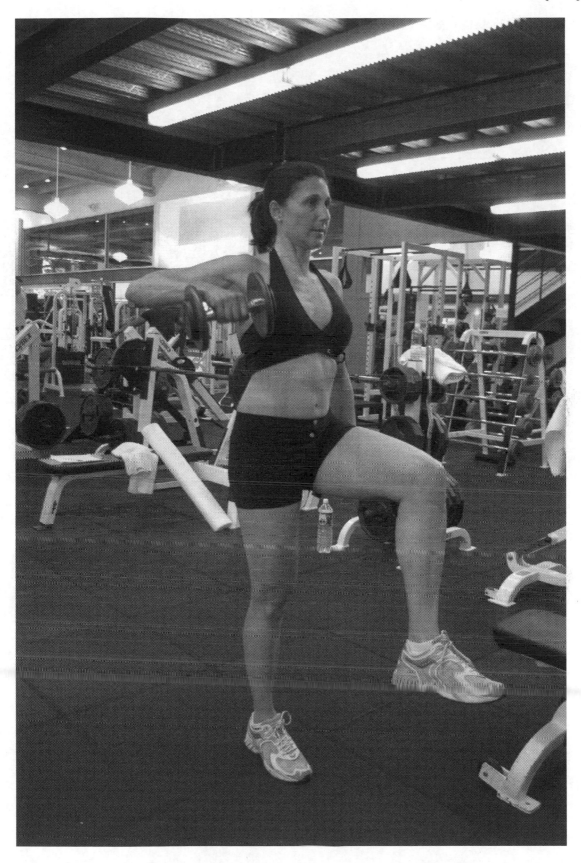

Then initiate the arm motion. Be sure to lead with the elbow as shown in figure 23B.

Dumbbell Bench Lunges.

This exercise is a way to improve on your traditional lunge.

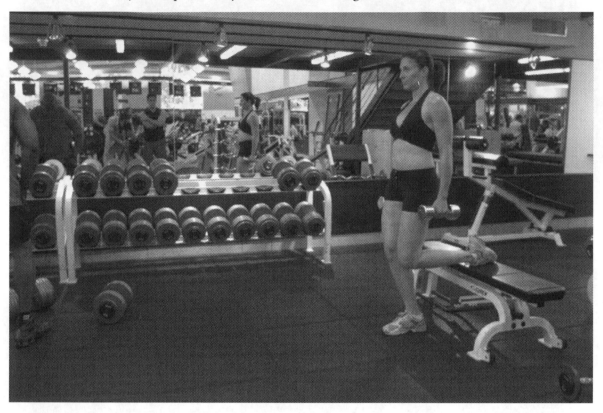

Picture 24a: Start with enough space to lunge forward and choose a comfortable weight. Start with one foot on the bench which is the same leg that will be lunging forward as shown in figure 24A.

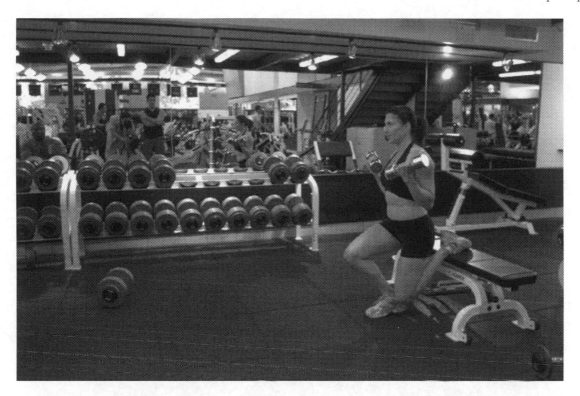

Picture 24B Begin to sit back approximating your heel to your butt but do not rest on the heel as shown in figure 24B.

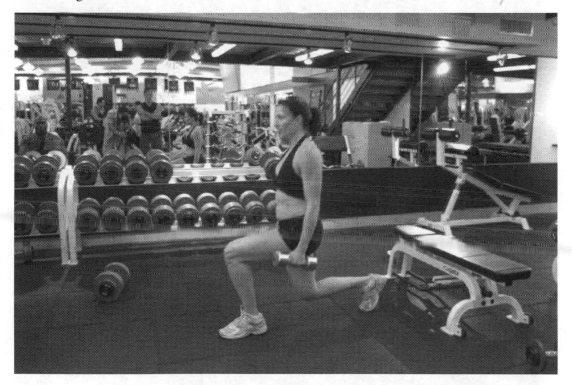

Picture 24 C Then begin to lunge forward with the same leg as shown in figure 24C. To increase difficulty add a bicep curl as shown in figure 24B.

Unilateral Dumbbell Core Press.

This exercise will isolate the chest muscles at the same time working the abdominal muscles. Position yourself half off the bench, lay your spine on the edge of the bench as shown in figure 25A. Maintain the opposite leg and hip up and at 90 degrees

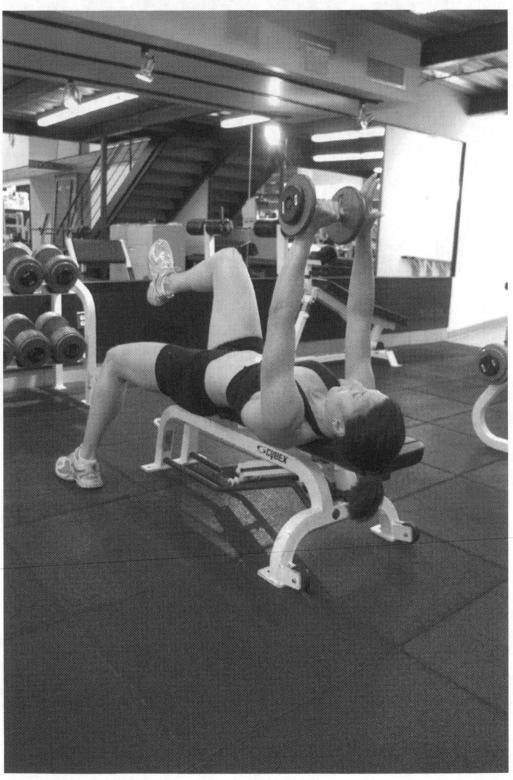

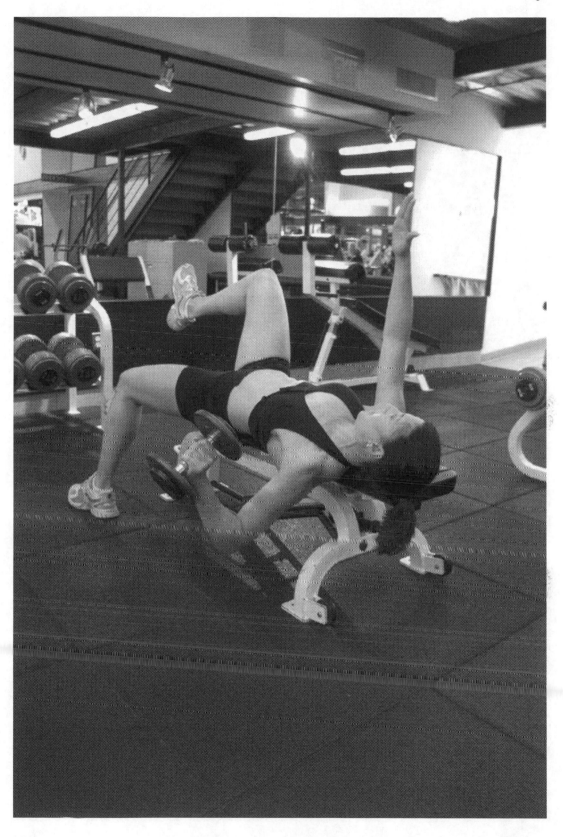

25B. Begin once your stable, to lower the dumbbell into a press. Be sure to feel the fibers stretching at the end of the motion

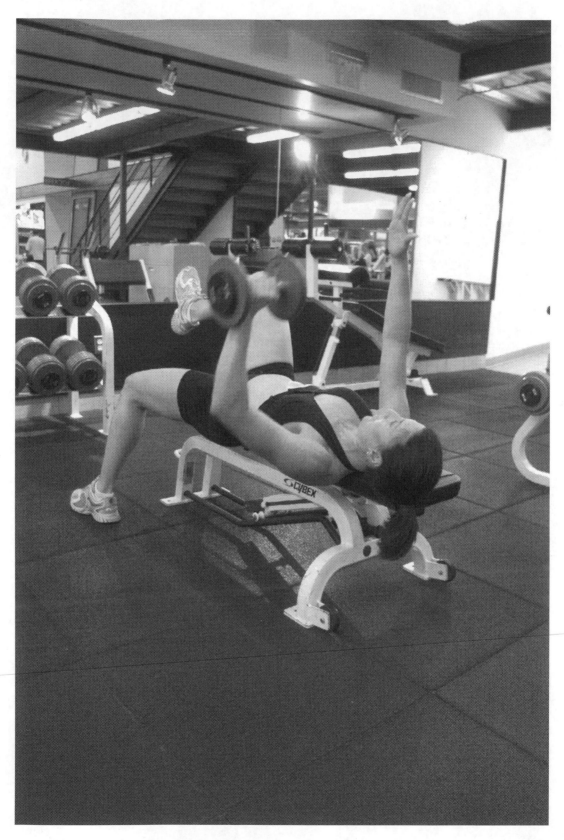

25c. Perform about 10-15 reps and switch over the other side of the bench to work the opposite side.

Sliding Core Pushup.

This exercise is a great way to incorporate a full body movement. Start off in a plank positon as shown in figure 26A. Lower yourself into a pushup as in figure 26B. Once coming out/up from the push-up position begin to pull in your legs at the same time utilizing the abdominal muscles. As shown in figure 26C.

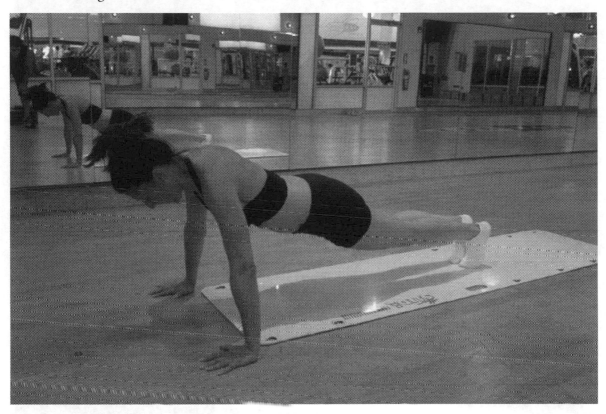

26a.

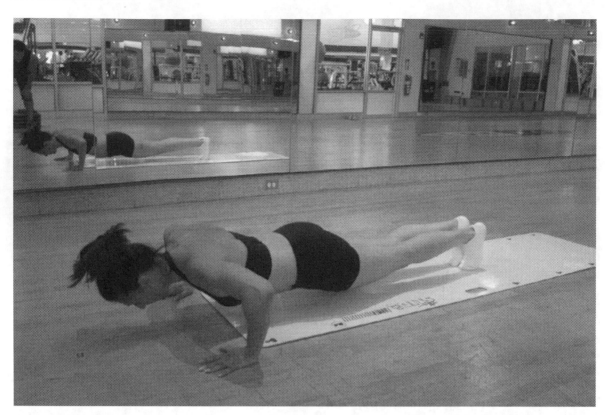

26b.

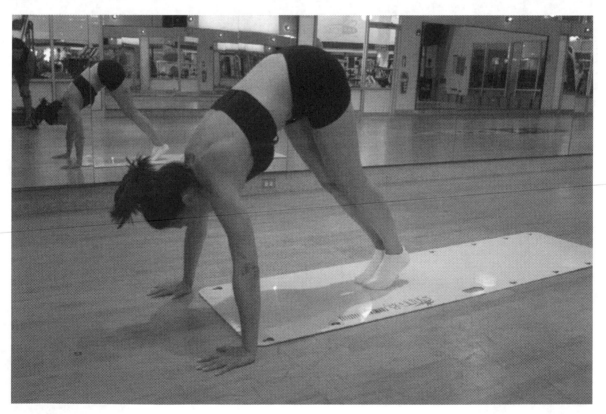

26c.

Side Step Jumps.

This exercise is a great way to get the heart rate up and build some lateral strength. Choose a step height which you feel comfortable jumping over. Start off in the position similar to a sprinters start , keep the inside foot up and generate your power through the other leg as shown in figure 27A.

Switch legs in mid air as in figure 27B and land the jump as shown in figure 27C.

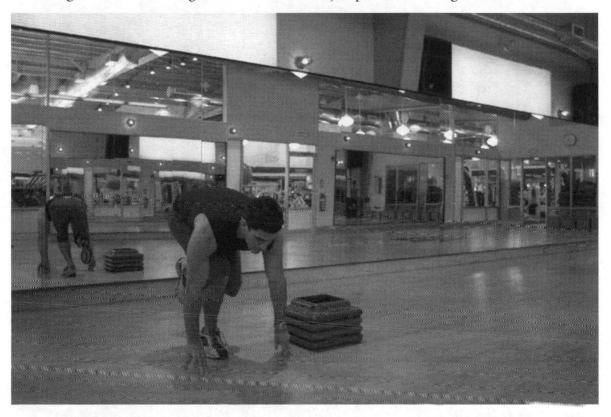

27a.

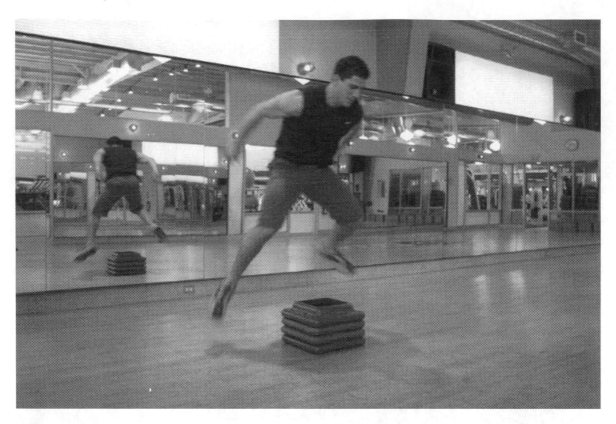

27b.

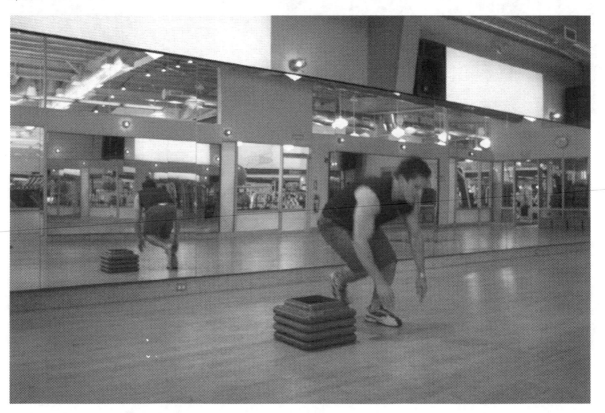

27c.

Ball Through Backs.

This is a great exercise to perform with a partner. This exercise will work on your reflexes and ablity to stabilize, maintaining a tight core while using the shoulders and low back muscles to throw the medicine ball back. Have your partner roll the ball to as shown in figure 28A. As the ball is approaching quickly react to grab the ball as in figure 28B. Then proceed to throw the ball over the opposite shoulder at your partner as in 28C. Repeat the exercise equally on both sides.

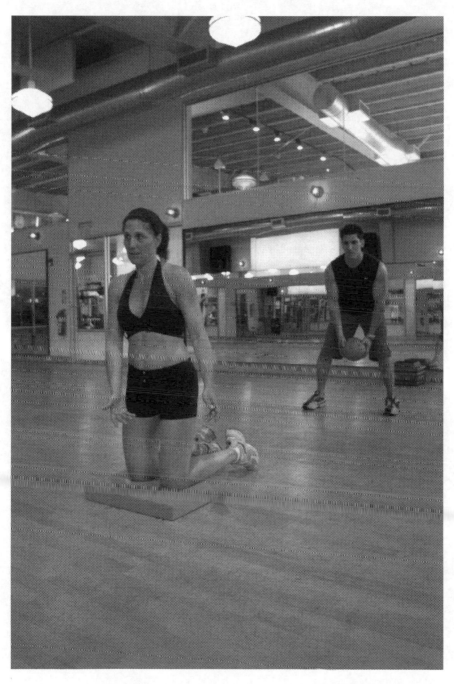

28a.

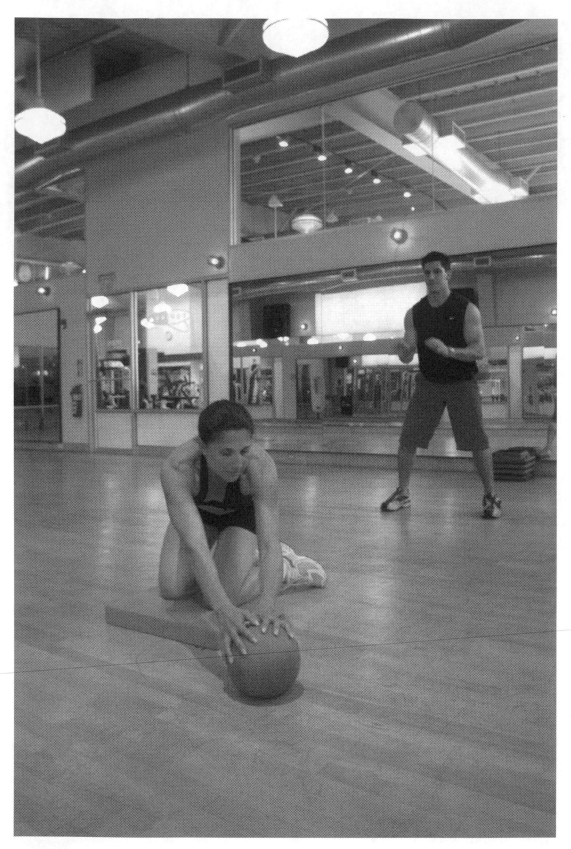

28b.

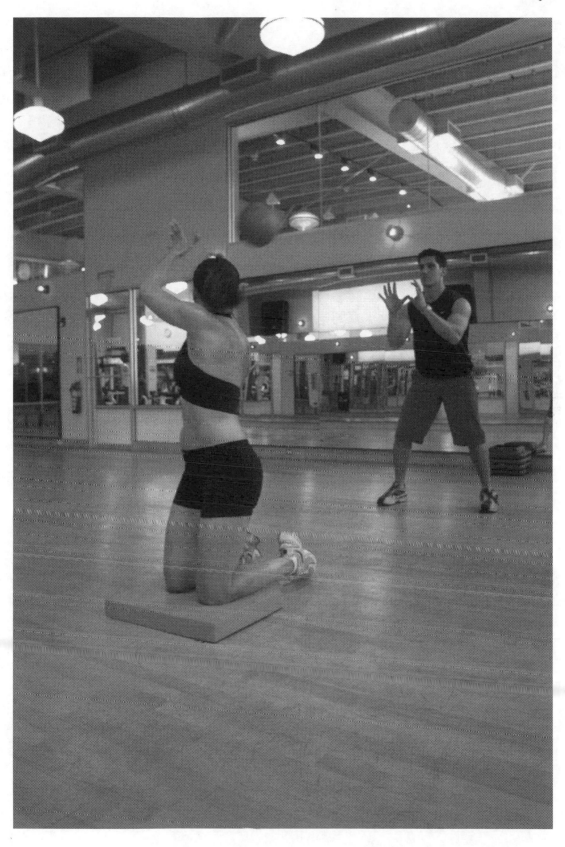

28c.

Bench Tri-cep Extensions.

This particular exercise will strengthen the triceps and at the same time the abdominals. Choose a weight which is comfortable but challenging, keep your legs straight and slightly elevated as in figure 29A. Begin to press the dumbbell up extending the arms and at the same time lift the legs as shown in figure 29B.

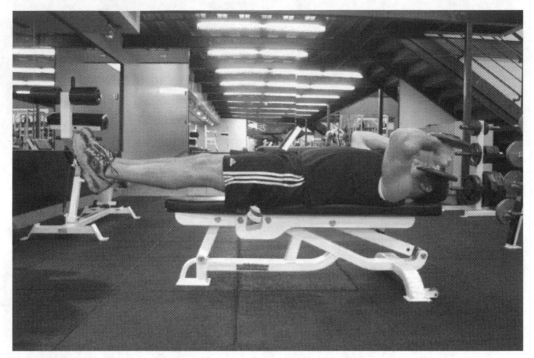

29a.

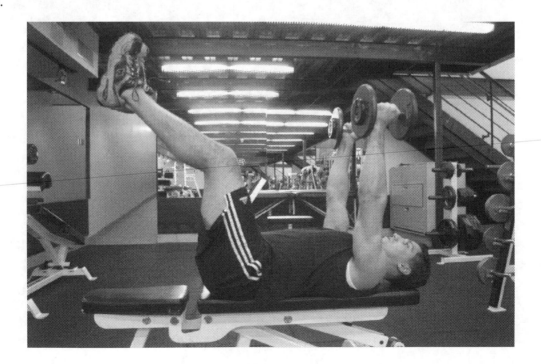

29b.

Hungarian Dead Lift.

This is a very challenging and effective exercise. A great way to improve stability and core strength. Performing this exercise helps with unilateral demanding sports. Initiate the exercise by standing on one leg holding a comfortable weight as in figure 30A. Begin to lower your body towards the ground slowly be sure to slightly bend the weight bearing knee. The opposite leg is kept straight to work the gluteal region. Lower the weight about 1 inch from the ground as shown in figure 30B. To add difficulty to this exercise, curl the weight at the top of the motion.

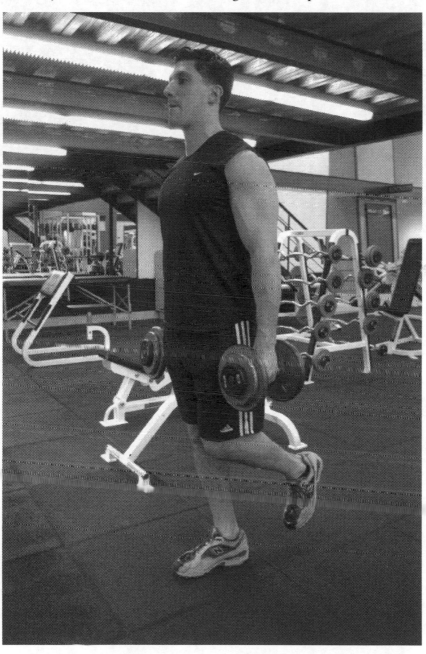

30a.

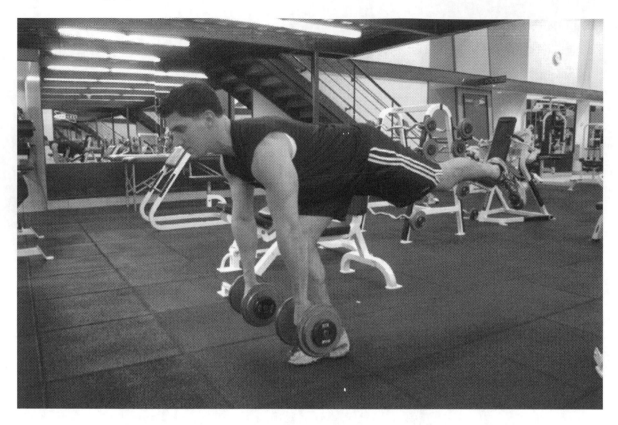

30b.

One Arm Upright Row.

This is a great alternative to the forbidden straight bar upright row. Use of the dumbbell allows the shoulder to move in its natural range of motion as opposed to the straight bar. Select a comfortable weight and perform the exercise while balancing on one leg as in figure 31A. When performing the row, lead with the elbow and remember to extend backwards at the end of the motion as in figure 31B.

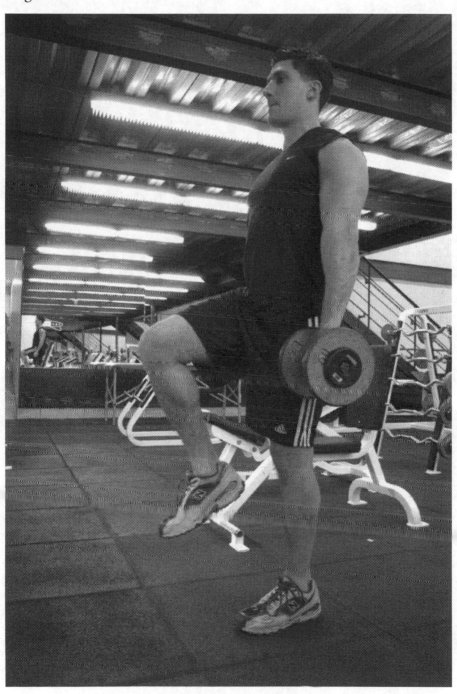

31a.

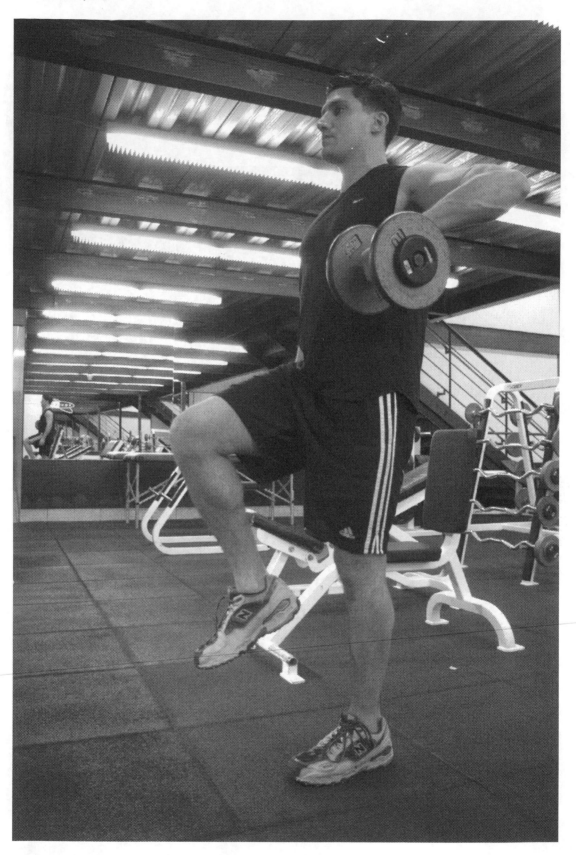

31b.

Hungarian Dead Lift On Half Foam Roller.

To further challenge your ability to balance and maintain a tight core use the half foam roller. The exercise is performed the same way as a normal Hungarian dead lift . Start in the upright position as shown in figure 32A. Slowly maintain control as you begin to lower yourself as in figure 32B. Once at end range hold the position for a few seconds challenging yourself further as in figure 32C.

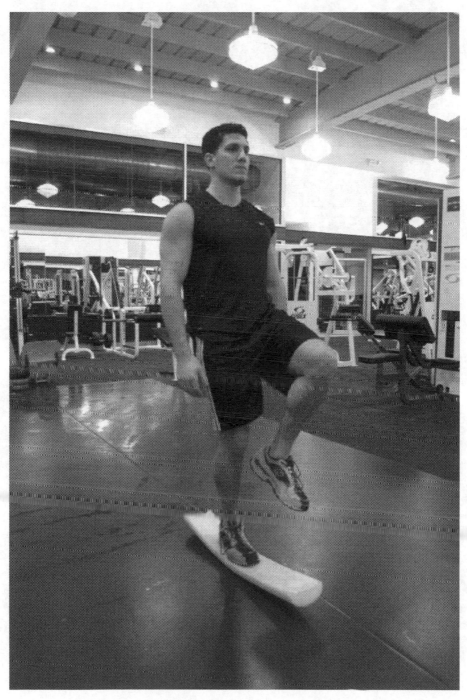

32a.

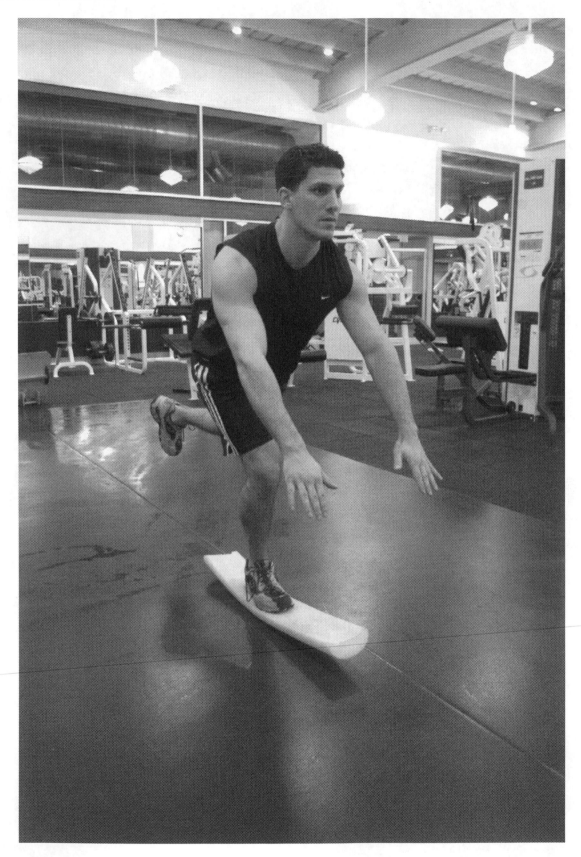

32b.

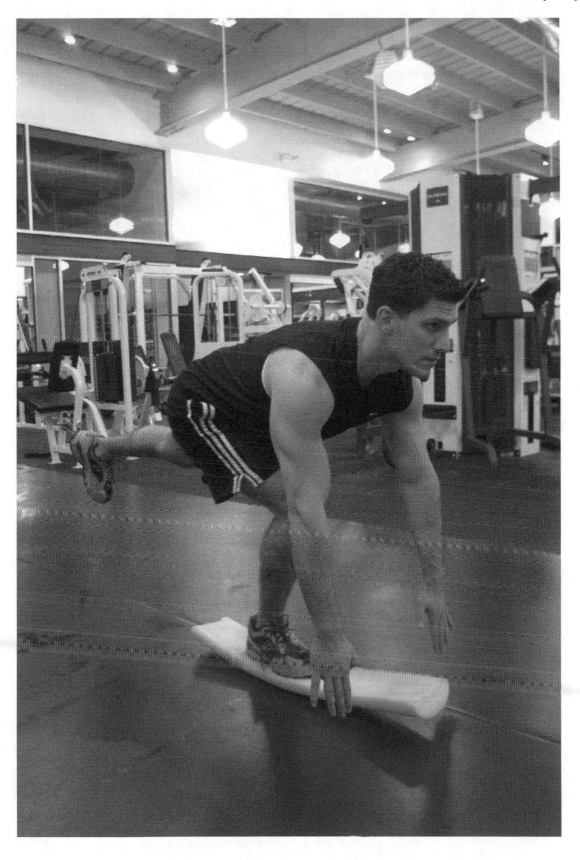

32c.

One Legged Half Foam Squat.

Once you have mastered the one legged squat without the foam roller and need a challenge this is the way to go. When performing the squat distribute your weight onto the heel maintain a tight core for increased stability as in figure 33A. Slowly lower yourself trying to maintain your balance as in figure 33B, if assistance is needed you may use a stick to lightly hold on to.

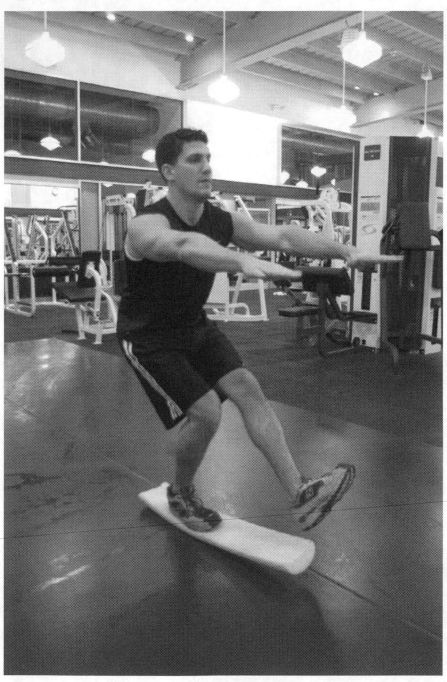

33a.

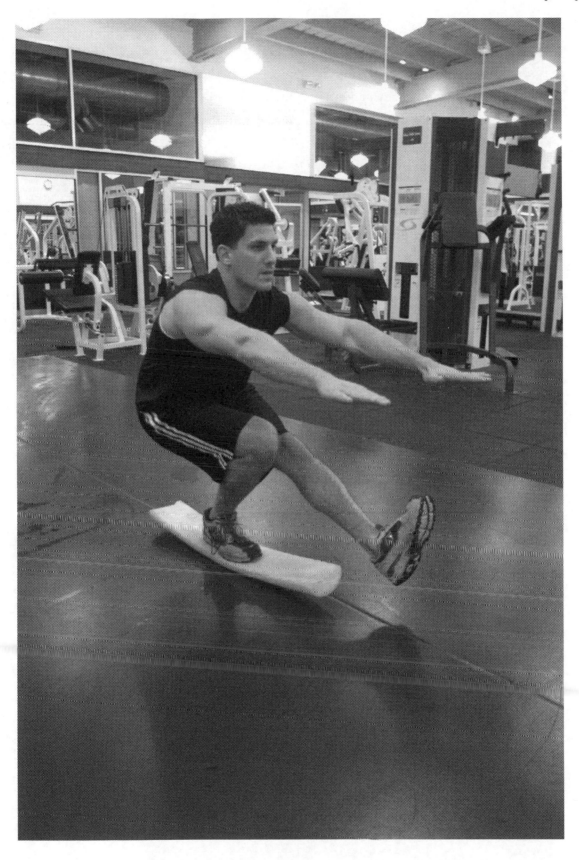

33b.

Core Ball Rotations.

If you are up to a challenge this is a great exercise for you. When performing this exercise, be sure there is something to grab on to for support. Climb onto the ball be and be sure to keep your abdominal muscles tight. Try to stand in an upright position and cross your arms for support as in picture 34a. Once you are stable and comfortable on the ball, begin rotations to each side as in figure 34b.

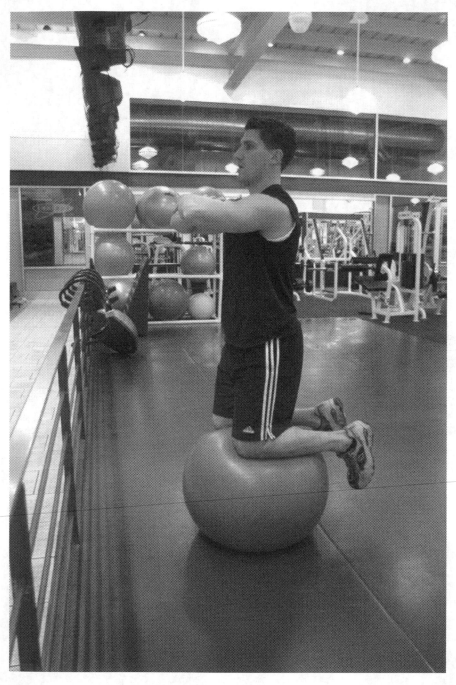

34a.

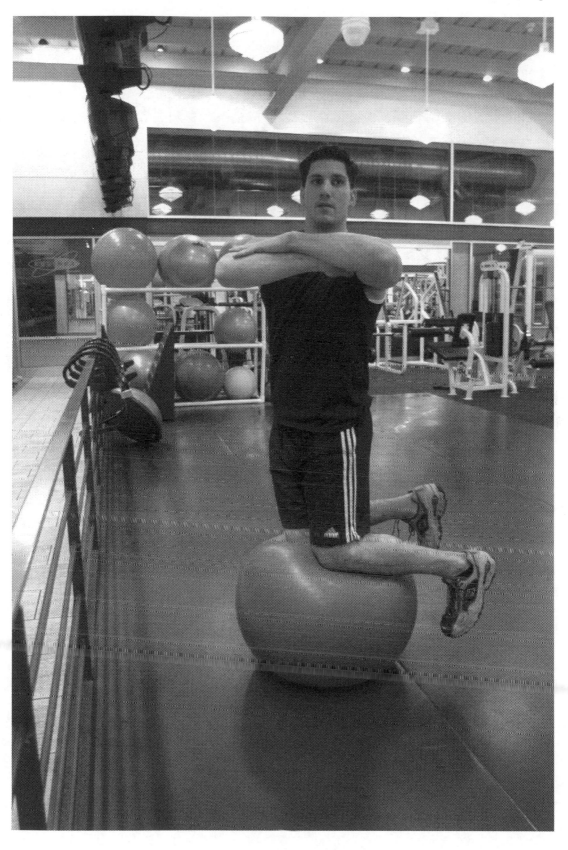

34b.

One Legged Ball Bridges

A bridge is a great way to isolate the gluteus and the abdominal muscles. Adding the ball to your bridge and performing it on one leg adds difficulty to this exercise. If it is too difficult perform it with both legs. When performing the exercise, stabilize with your arms. Extend one leg up in the air while stabilizing on the ball with the other as in figure 35a. Perform the exercise by lifting the pelvis up into the air as in figure 35b.

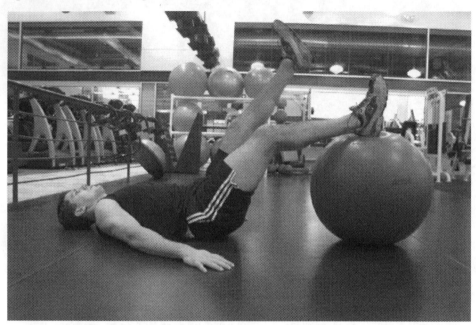

35a.

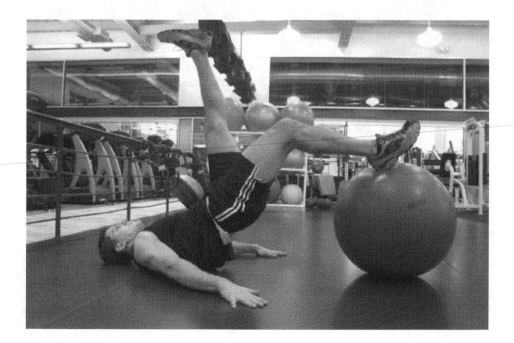

35b.

Seated Medicine Ball Rotations.

For those of you whom suffer from back pain this is the exercise for you. Select a excercise ball which is appropriate for your height. A good way to tell is when seated on the ball, your hips and knees should appear to be flexed at a 90 degree angle. Hold a medicine ball directly in front of you; choose a comfortable weight. Lift one foot up in the air while balancing on the other as in figure 36a. Once you have sustained your balance slowly initiate your movements by rotating to the side from the waist up as in figure 36b.

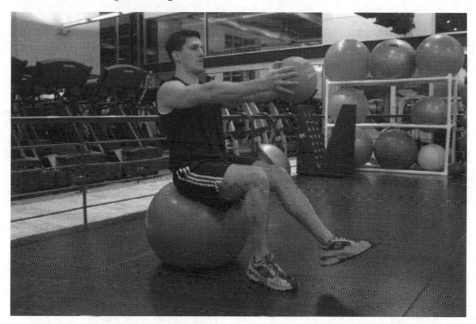

36a.

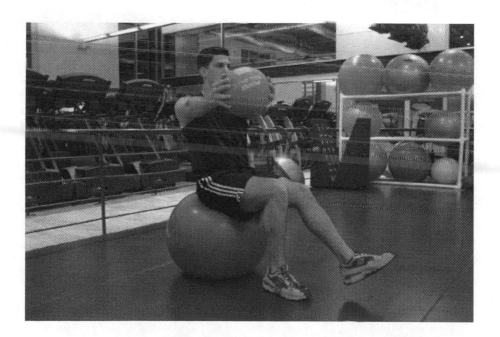

36b.

Dead Weight Push Ups.

Here's a push-up which challenges your core strength directly. Starting from a relaxed position will require you to engage your core muscles each time you attempt the pushup. The starting position is shown in figure 37A.

37a: Be sure your hand positioning is low and tight. I like to keep my palm in line with the bottom of my breast bone. Once in position begin to initiate the movement as in figure 37A. Be sure to keep your back straight.37B

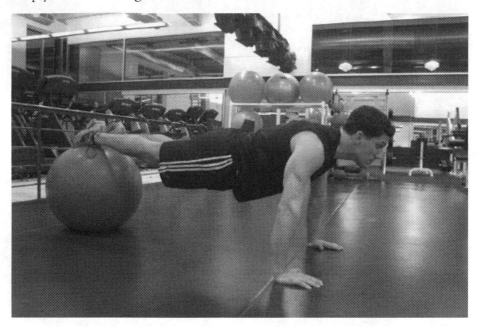

37a.

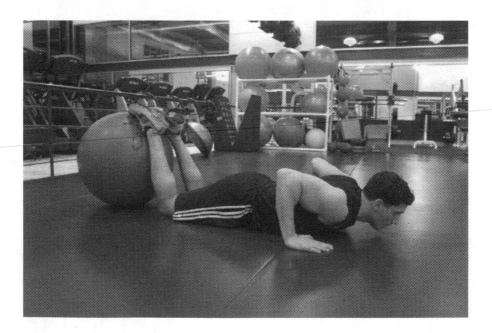

37b.

Half Foam Medicine Ball Squats.

Squatting on a half foam roll is a great way to learn how to squat properly. If you are not distributing your weight properly, you will roll off the edge.

38a: Choose a medicine ball for assisted balance and assume the starting position.

38b: When squatting, be sure not to emphasize all your weight forward. Try to sit back on your heels holding your balance as in figure 38B.

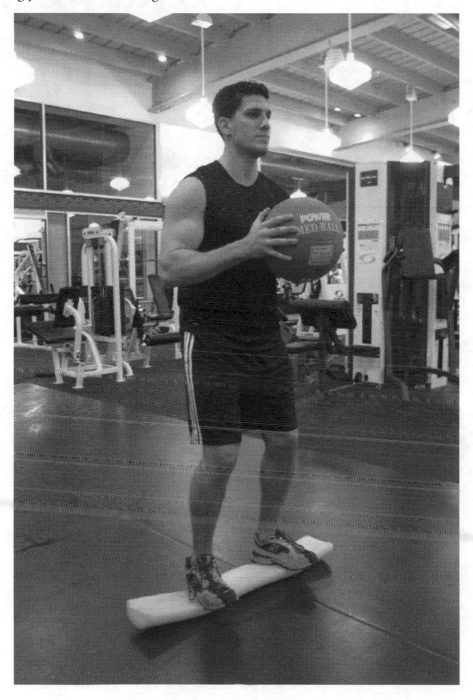

38a.

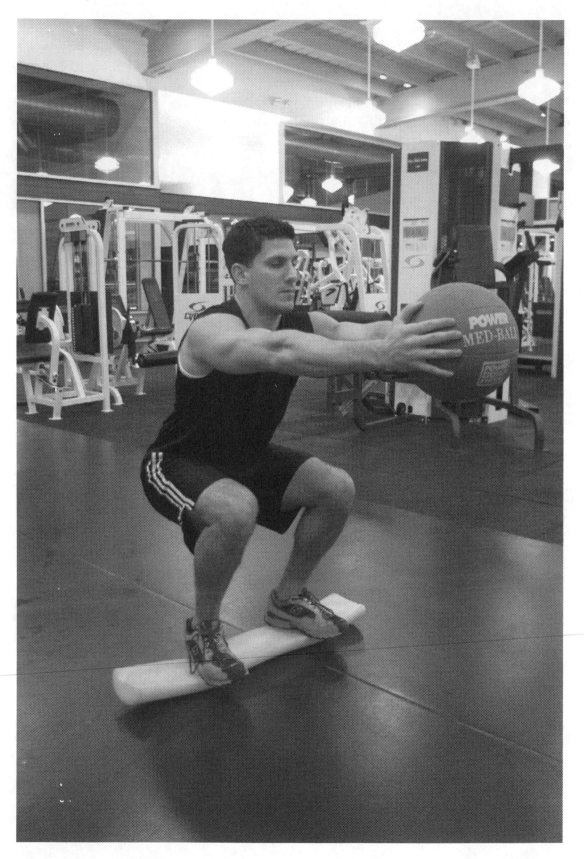

38b.

Physio Ball Fly's.

This is for those whom have a strong chest and stable core. Choose two balls of equal height and size.

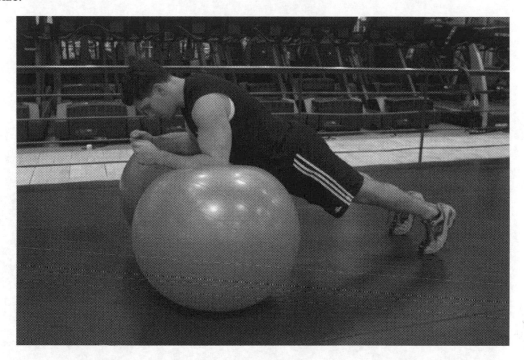

39a: Begin by resting the elbows into the balls as in figure 39A.

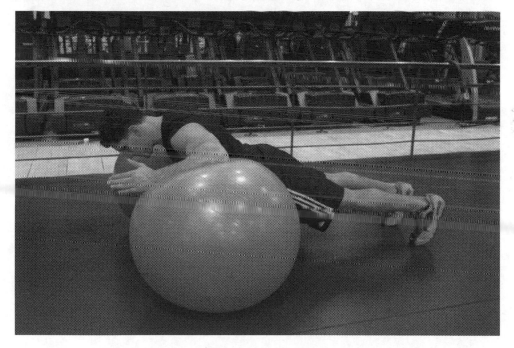

39b: Keep the legs straight and the stomach tight. Slowly lower your chest to the ground and be sure to maintain control to avoid any injury.

Rotational Ball Raises.

This exercise focuses on spinal stabilization in a neutral pelvis position.

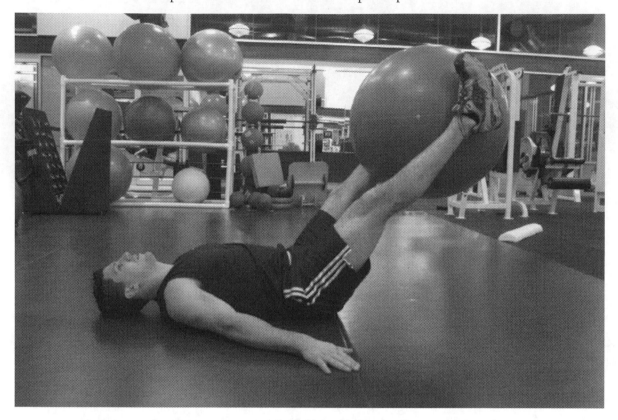

40a: Squeeze the ball between your legs engaging the adductors and lift as shown in this picture.

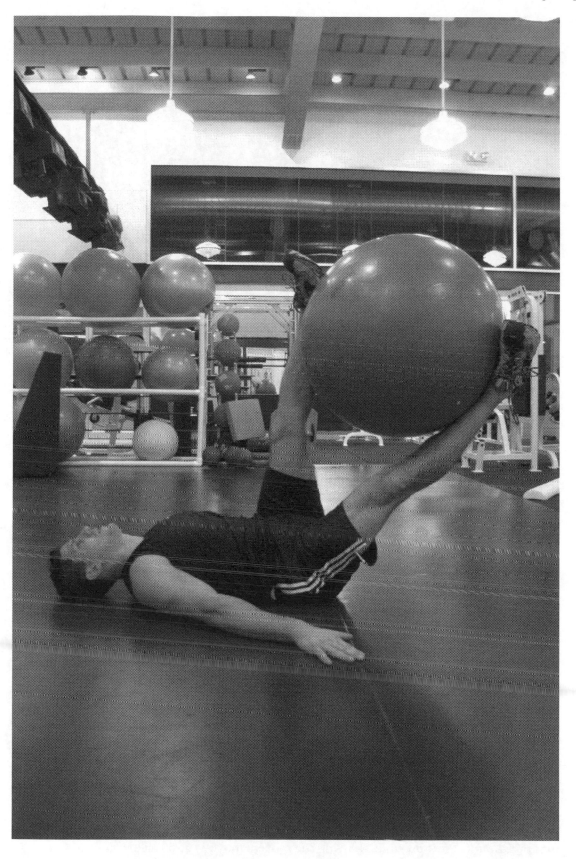

40b: Once you have reached a comfortable range, begin to twist to the side.

Dead Bug.

This is a great exercise when it comes to strengthening the lower back. The key to performing this exercise is control and speed.

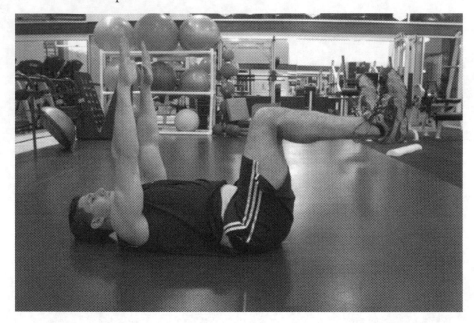

41a: Assume the position as shown in figure 41A. The goal is to hold your joints at 90 degrees (shoulders, hips, knees and ankles). In relation to the lower back, try to depress the small of your back into the mat.

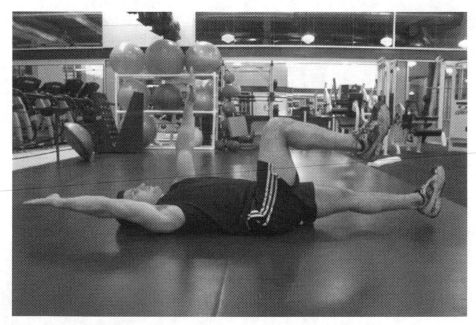

41b: Once in this position begin to initiate movement by lowering the opposite arm and leg to the mat but do not rest if possible. During the movement you must make a conscious effort not to move the stationary arm and leg. Proceed by alternating movements.

Coordination and strength are tested here.

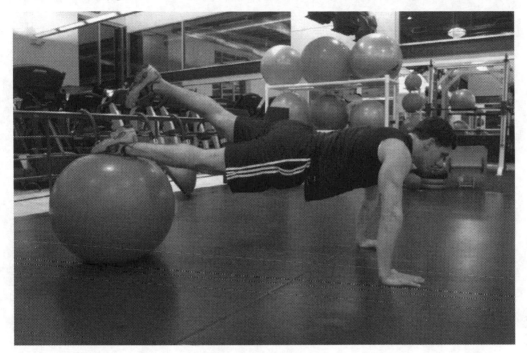

42a: Choose a ball of appropriate height for your body. Assume the position shown in figure 42A and be sure to keep your abdominal tight. Lift one leg up and stabilize with your other.

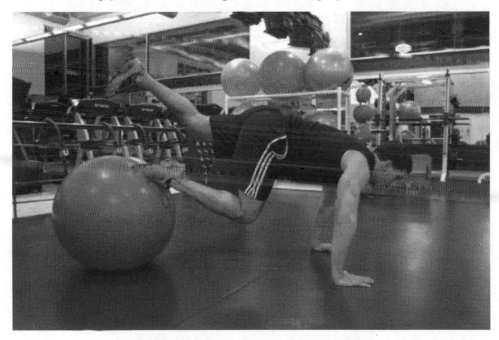

42b: Start the exercise by bringing the stabilizing leg to your chest while the other leg remains up.

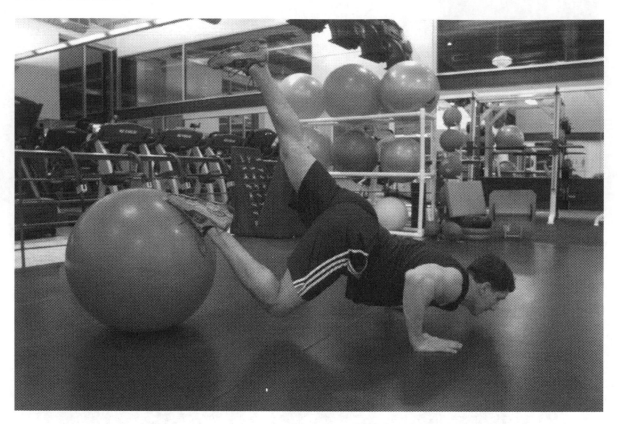

42c: As you approach the end of your range, perform a push up. Repeat the movement slowly and controlled to avoid any injury.

Ball Hip Hinge

This is a great way to work those hip flexors and the abdominals.

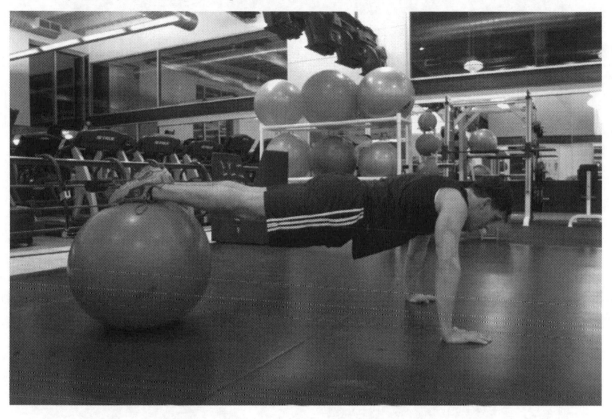

43a: Select a ball of appropriate height and assume a plank position.

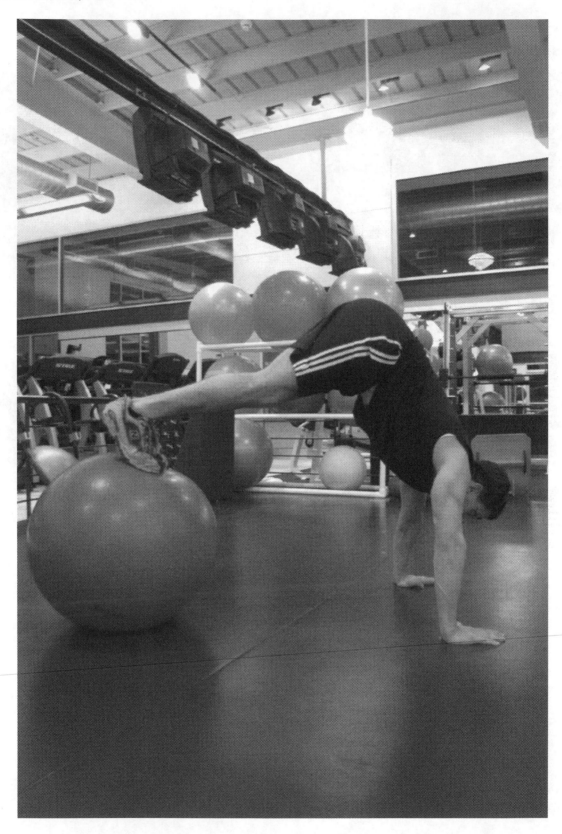

43b: Begin to flex at the hips by bringing the ball forwards. Be sure to hold the knees straight which helps to isolate the abdominals.

One Legged Ball Bridge.

Ball bridging is a great way to strengthen your core as well as your lower back area. To further challenge yourself try to isolate one leg.

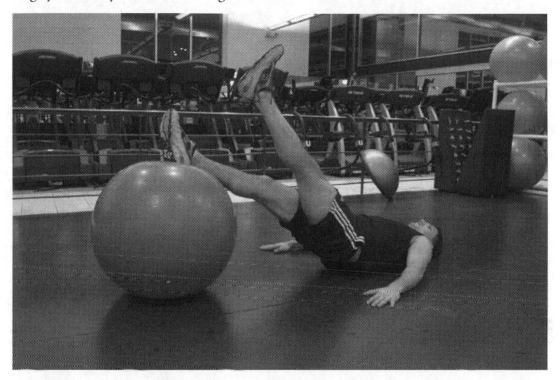

44a: Assume the position as shown in this figure. Keep the pelvis raised off the mat.

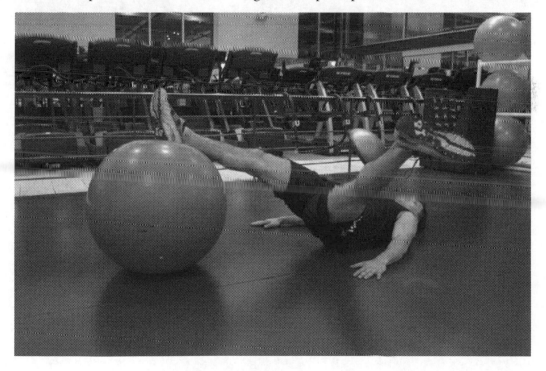

44b: Begin to abduct or extend your leg to the side.

Ball Pelvis Rotation.

Add a little twist to your ball bridge!

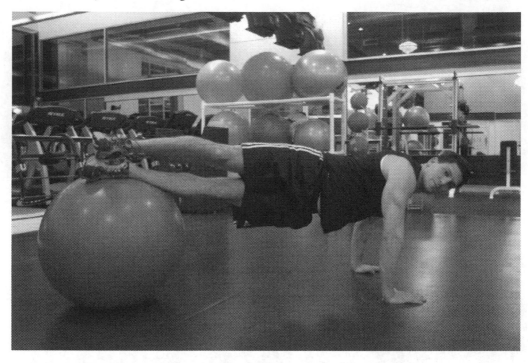

45a: Assume a plank position with the lower torso rotated to one side as shown. Be sure to hold your abdominals tightly.

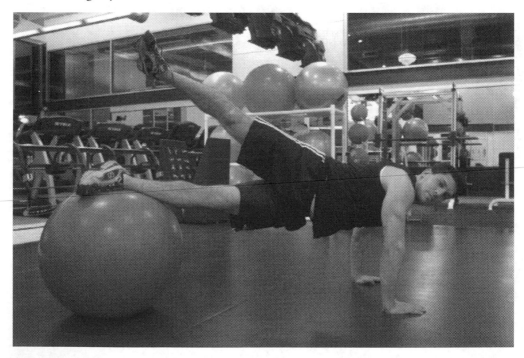

45b: In the starting position begin to abduct the superior leg. Repeat about 10-15 reps and then switch to the other side.

Dumbbell Torso Rotations.

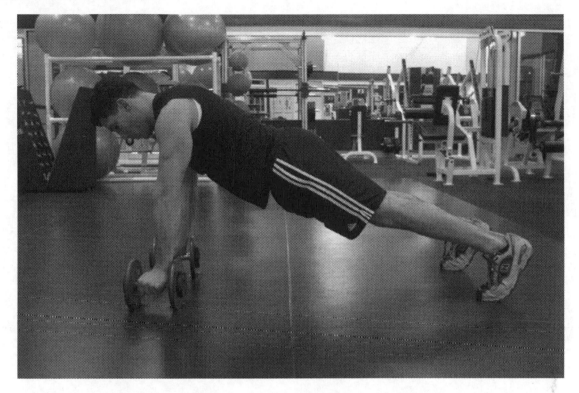

46a: Select a weight with which you have no problem doing a rear deltoid row with. Assume a plank position using the dumbbell as your foundation.

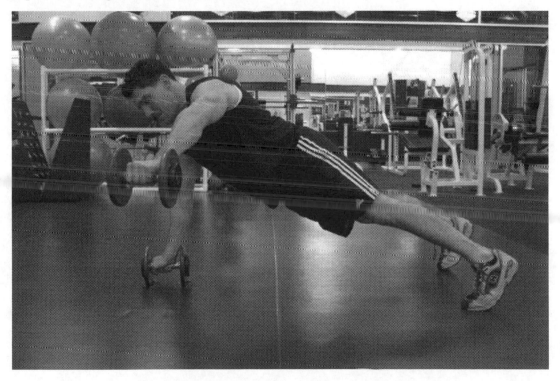

46b: Slowly begin to rotate to the side lifting and leading with the dumbbell.

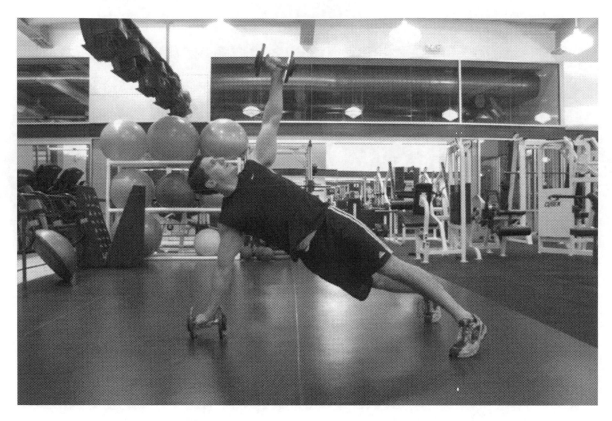

46c: Continue to lift the dumbbell until about 180 degrees of torso rotation as shown in picture above.

Side Bends.

This exercise strengthens the lower back and love handle region. If you have shoulder issues you might want to skip this exercise because of the direct weight bearing on the shoulder.

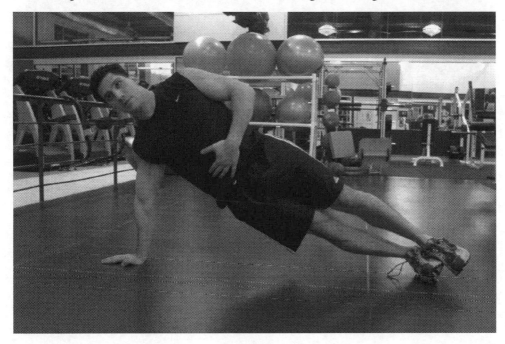

47a: Position yourself as shown in figure 47A. Be sure to keep your shoulder, hip and feet in a straight line.

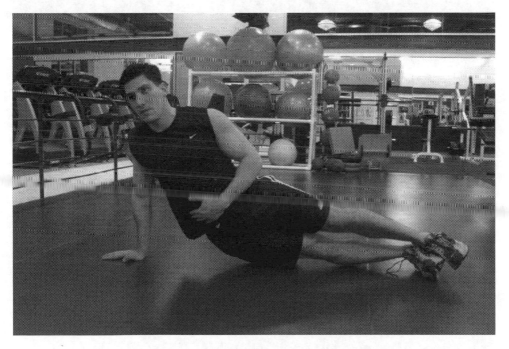

47b: Begin to lower yourself slowly to the mat to the point where there is a stretch. Then proceed to return to the starting position.

Pelvis Ball Bridges.

This is a great way to work the glutes, hamstrings and abdominal region.

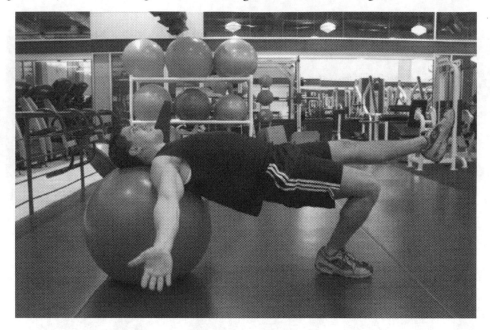

48a: From the sitting position roll yourself down and forward on the ball resting your shoulders on the ball. From this position hold your arms out for increased stability and lift one leg up as in figure 49A.

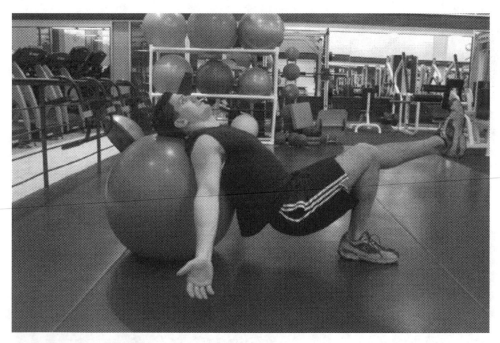

48b: Once in this position and stable, lower your pelvis to the ground slowly about 2-3 inches off the ground. Hold for about 2-3 seconds then begin to lift by pushing through the stabilizing leg returning to starting position.

Ball Low Back Extensions.

Use this exercise to build the lower back musculature and to create an upright posture.

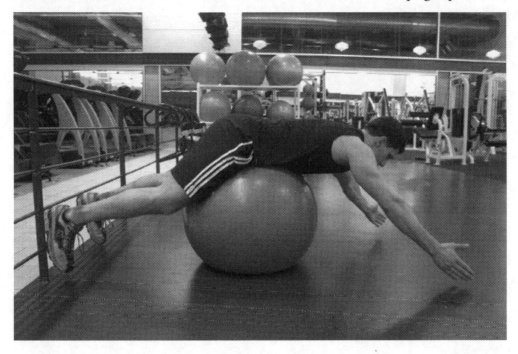

49a: Begin by resting your anterior pelvis directly on the ball as shown in figure 49A. For decreased difficulty anchor feet against the wall or whatever seems appropriate from your environment.

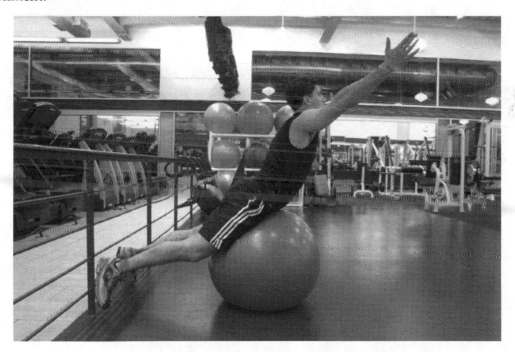

49b: Begin to extend to the ceiling leading with the arms; it is very important to hold the shoulder blades pinched when performing this movement.

NOTES

SPECIFIC TRAINING PROGRAMS

Football Off Season
Perform exercises 5, 6, 8, 10, 17, 18, 21, 25, 27, 30, 37, 39.

Skiing/Snowboarding
Perform exercises 5, 10, 11, 12, 13, 14, 16, 21.

Tennis
Perform exercises 8, 9, 11, 16, 18, 22, 27, 45.

Soccer
Perform exercises 10, 32, 33, 38, 40, 43, 44, 45.

Golf
Perform exercises 5, 7, 12, 17, 30, 40.

Hockey
Perform exercises 16, 21, 33, 37, 40.

Baseball
Perform exercises 4, 8, 10, 11, 25, 30.

Figure Skating
Perform exercises 1, 5, 10, 16, 21, 44, 45.

Basketball
Perform exercises 4, 10, 11, 12, 13, 14, 24, 27.